化学工业出版社"十四五"普通高等教育规划教材

普通高等教育药学类系列教材

石油和化工行业"十四五"规划教材

药物化学实验（双语）

（第二版）

李　雯　郑一超　陆小云　主编

尤启冬　主审

Experiments of Medicinal Chemistry

化学工业出版社

·北京·

Introduction

Experiments of Medicinal Chemistry (*Second Edition*) mainly includes five parts: chemical drug synthesis experiments, experimental report templates, commonly used instruments, reference answers to thinking questions and boiling points and dielectric constants of commonly used solvents. In the part of chemical drug synthesis experiments, 19 drugs were arranged in the order from basic to comprehensive. This textbook emphasizes the relationship between theoretical teaching and experiment of pharmaceutical chemistry, and pays attention to training students' experimental ability and scientific research quality. In an effort to adapt to the contemporary trend of internationalization of higher education, this textbook is compiled in a Chinese-English bilingual system.

This textbook is suitable for the experimental teaching of pharmacy students (including foreign students) in medical colleges and universities.

内容简介

《药物化学实验（双语）(Experiments of Medicinal Chemistry)》（第二版）主要包括化学药物合成实验、实验报告模板、常规仪器、思考题参考答案以及常用溶剂的沸点和介电常数五个部分。化学药物合成实验部分按照基础操作到综合实验的顺序安排了 19 个药物的合成实验，强调了药物化学理论教学与实验的关联，关注学生实验能力和科研素质的培养。为适应高等教育国际化的趋势，本教材采用中英双语体系编写。

《药物化学实验（双语）(Experiments of Medicinal Chemistry)》（第二版）适用于高等医药院校药学类专业学生（包括留学生）的实验教学。

图书在版编目（CIP）数据

药物化学实验 = Experiments of Medicinal
Chemistry：英汉对照 / 李雯，郑一超，陆小云主编.
2 版. -- 北京：化学工业出版社，2025. 3. --（化学工
业出版社"十四五"普通高等教育规划教材）. -- ISBN
978-7-122-47119-2

Ⅰ. R914-33

中国国家版本馆 CIP 数据核字第 2025YZ3625 号

责任编辑：孙钦炜　褚红喜　宋林青　　装帧设计：关　飞
责任校对：宋　玮

出版发行：化学工业出版社
　　　　　（北京市东城区青年湖南街 13 号　邮政编码 100011）
印　　装：河北鑫兆源印刷有限公司
787mm×1092mm　1/16　印张 15¾　字数 398 千字
2025 年 3 月北京第 2 版第 1 次印刷

购书咨询：010-64518888　　　售后服务：010-64518899
网　　址：http：//www. cip. com. cn

Experiments of Medicinal Chemistry
(Second Edition)

Editor in chief

Wen Li（School of pharmaceutical sciences，Zhengzhou University）

Yichao Zheng（School of pharmaceutical sciences，Zhengzhou University）

Xiaoyun Lu（School of pharmacy，Jinan University）

Associate editors in chief

En Zhang（School of pharmaceutical sciences，Zhengzhou University）

Kai Sun（School of pharmaceutical sciences，Zhengzhou University）

Lina Ding（School of pharmaceutical sciences，Zhengzhou University）

Yajing Chen（School of pharmaceutical sciences，Zhengzhou University）

Reviewer in chief

Qidong You（China Pharmaceutical University）

Other Editors

Xiaoyu Chang（School of pharmaceutical sciences，Zhengzhou University）

Yingchao Duan（Xinxiang Medical University）

Yonggang Meng（School of pharmaceutical sciences，Zhengzhou University）

Peng Sang（School of pharmaceutical sciences，Zhengzhou University）

Yan Shi（School of pharmaceutical sciences，Zhengzhou University）

Saiyang Zhang（School of basic medicine，Zhengzhou University）

药物化学实验（双语）
（第二版）

主　编

李　雯　（郑州大学药学院）

郑一超　（郑州大学药学院）

陆小云　（暨南大学药学院）

副主编

张　恩　（郑州大学药学院）

孙　凯　（郑州大学药学院）

丁丽娜　（郑州大学药学院）

陈亚静　（郑州大学药学院）

主　审

尤启冬　（中国药科大学）

其他编者（以姓氏首字母排序）

常晓宇　（郑州大学药学院）

段迎超　（新乡医学院）

孟勇刚　（郑州大学药学院）

桑　鹏　（郑州大学药学院）

石　岩　（郑州大学药学院）

张赛扬　（郑州大学基础医学院）

序 一

新药创制推动了个性化治疗和精准医疗的发展，是解决难治性疾病和罕见病的有效措施，也是应对突发疫情和公共卫生危机的关键手段。在面临如新型冠状病毒（COVID-19）感染这样的全球性疫情时，新药研发能够迅速提供有效的治疗手段，减轻医疗系统的压力，保障人民生命健康。

新药创制涉及从基础科学研究到临床应用的多个环节，是一个复杂且高度知识密集型的过程，在这个过程中，药物化学实验的知识和技能为新药的发现提供了坚实的化学基础，贯穿于新药研发的各个阶段，在药物设计、先导化合物的合成、化学结构改造和优化、合成工艺优化、揭示药物作用机制以及质量控制的每一个环节，都发挥着至关重要的作用。

实验，是科学探索的基石，也是药学人才培养的关键环节。这本《药物化学实验（双语）》（第二版）教材坚持以双语体系编写，提供了19个药物的合成实验，涉及非甾体抗炎药物、局部麻醉药物、合成抗菌药物、抗癫痫药物、抗胆碱酯酶药物、钙通道阻滞剂类药物、抗病毒药物、抗肿瘤药物的合成，包含了丰富的反应类型，以图片、视频、虚拟仿真实验等数字化形式融入了大量的药物合成操作、作用机制、化合物活性评价方法等知识，也提供了药物的含量测定方法，体现了药物化学实验课程的独立性、系统性和科学性，又充分考虑到各门实验课程之间的联系与衔接。此外，本教材重视编者的科研成果向教学的转化，紧跟药物化学领域的最新研究成果和技术进展，体现了时效性与前沿性，既重视学生基本实验技能的拓展，也满足学生创新创业能力培养的需求，同时使学生在实验教学过程中，加深对我国自主研发新药的认识，增强民族自豪感。

希望这本《药物化学实验（双语）》（第二版）教材能够为培养更多具有国际视野、创新精神和实践能力的药学人才贡献力量。

常俊标

2025 年 1 月

序 二

为了适应高等教育全球化发展的重要趋势，充分利用和发挥我国优质的教育资源，加强国际教育和教学交流，注重培养具有国际视野和跨文化交流能力的人才，编写和出版我国双语教材有着重要的价值和意义。

2019 年，郑州大学药学院根据留学生教学和中国学生双语教学的需求，开展实验教学研究和改革，编写和出版了《药物化学实验双语教程（Experiments of Medicinal Chemistry）》。经过 5 年的教学和实践，编者在总结经验的基础上，对该教材进行改进，并引入数字化资源，编写了《药物化学实验（双语）》(第二版)。与第一版教材相比，本书的主要特色包括：

（1）新增地平类药物、肽类药物、核苷类药物、替尼类药物的合成实验，丰富了药物的结构类型和合成方法。

（2）增加 Pd/TB-COF 负载型纳米催化剂的合成和苯佐卡因的合成的虚拟仿真实验，丰富了实验教学方式。且在此部分增加了化合物的核磁共振氢谱解析，以培养学生的结构确证能力。

（3）在实验装置部分，每个化合物的合成均增加了合成装置的实景照片，以方便学生以直观的方式尽快理解实验操作过程，减少因语言问题造成的理解障碍。

（4）教材中实验三至实验八、实验十二，均以二维码形式提供了实验操作的视频资料。

（5）在每个药物的背景知识部分，增加了化合物活性评价方法，以培养学生结构-活性关联的意识。

（6）在每个药物的合成实验中，新增了药物含量的测定方法，以培养学生药品质量的观念。

本教材的内容体现了药物设计-化学合成-结构确证-活性评价-含量分析等知识的综合性，是创新型人才培养的一种积极尝试。期待从事药物化学实验教育的同行们在实验的教学上大胆改革，共同促进药物化学实验双语教学的发展。

尤启冬

2024 年 10 月

序（第一版）

随着我国教育国际化进程的发展，高等教育的国际化已由原有的单纯"走出去"，逐渐转变为"走出去"和"招进来"相结合的模式。越来越多的外国留学生，特别是"一带一路"沿线国家和亚非等国的外国留学生到中国来学习。但我国双语教材的建设速度与日益增多的留学生发展趋势不能同步，因此，进行双语教材的编写和推广使用工作有着非常重要的价值和意义。

郑州大学药学院根据药学专业中国学生双语教学的需求和留学生教学的需求，开展实验教学研究，编写和出版了《药物化学实验双语教程（Experiments of Medicinal Chemistry)》。

该教材重视加强学生科研能力的培养，是作者针对国内学生和留学生的实际情况，分析现行各版本教材的内容和特点，博采众家所长而编写的教材，具有以下特色：

（1）在实验原理部分，增加主要原料和产物的物性常数，包括分子量、熔点、沸点和溶解度等参数，以培养学生通过思考和实验操作，触类旁通，提高解决问题的能力，且配以图表便于理解。

（2）增加安全提醒内容，以预防部分学生对危险化学品的错误使用而造成严重后果。

（3）在实验操作方面，增加实验装置图示，以方便学生以直观的方式尽快理解实验操作过程。

（4）增加药物受体和配体相互作用的计算机模拟图示，体现了实验课程对理论课程知识的综合应用和拓展。

（5）为培养学生对实验现象规范记录和结果分析能力，本教材提供了实例并提出了具体的要求，使学生进一步联系理论，做出分析比较。

（6）增加思考题的参考答案，给学生一些提示，方便更好地理解实验相关问题，有助于培养学生的学习兴趣。

相信本教材的出版能够促进我国药物化学实验双语教学的发展。

尤启冬

（国家实验教学示范中心联席会药学学科组组长、国家教学名师）

2019 年 3 月

前　言

2019 年，全国高等教育药学类规划教材《药物化学实验双语教程（Experiments of Medicinal Chemistry)》第一版出版。该教材对药学类专业学生，尤其是对留学生的教学发挥了重要作用。为进一步适应国家和社会对创新型药学人才培养的需求和本科教学国际化的发展趋势，我们在第一版教材的基础上进行修订，编写了《药物化学实验（双语）（Experiments of Medicinal Chemistry)》第二版。

与第一版相比，本教材保留原有的 10 个实验，新增有关地平类药物、肽类药物、核苷类药物、替尼类药物合成的 9 个实验，总计为 19 个实验。此外，本教材还增加了苯佐卡因合成的虚拟仿真实验（若需要开展该虚拟仿真实验，请通过邮件形式联系编者，liwen@zzu.edu.cn），丰富了药物的结构类别、合成方法和学习方式。本教材中实验三至实验八、实验十二，均以二维码形式提供了数字化内容，主要为实验操作演示视频资料。更为重要的是，新增的实验除了包含近年来新上市的药物，也涉及具有我国自主知识产权的创新药物和编者的科研成果。

此次修订在每个药物的背景知识部分，增加了化合物活性评价方法，以加深学生对结构-活性关系的理解；在每个药物的实验原理部分，增加了知识点的内容，以帮助学生理解和掌握学习重点；在每个药物的合成实验中，新增了药物含量的测定方法，以培养学生药品质量意识。在苯佐卡因合成的虚拟仿真实验中，增加了化合物的核磁共振氢谱解析，以培养学生的结构确证能力。本教材的内容既重视对学生药物合成能力的培养，也充分体现了药物设计-化学合成-结构确证-活性评价-含量分析等知识的综合性，有利于培养学生灵活运用药学综合知识的能力，是创新型人才培养的一种积极尝试。

本教材中，实验一、实验二由李雯和郑一超编写，实验七、实验八、实验九和实验十四由李雯编写，实验三、实验四由陈亚静编写，实验五由丁丽娜编写，实验六由张恩编写，实验十由孙凯编写，实验十一由段迎超编写，实验十二由郑一超编写，实验十三由张赛扬编写，实验十五由桑鹏编写，实验十六由石岩编写，实验十七由孟勇刚编写，实验十八由常晓宇编写，实验十九由陆小云编写。本教材由尤启冬审定。教材中药物分子和靶标的作用机制部分由丁丽娜及研究生阎影、马超亚、王志正、高琦冰、孙旭东、杨晶、刘欢和王兵丽等借助 MOE 软件作图及编写，教材中有关药物活性评价方式的部分由郑一超进行编写。留学中国的博士研究生 Muhammad Zeeshan、研究生朱林元参与了本教材的语言修订工作。

本教材采用中英双语体系编写，可用于高等医药院校药学类专业学生（包括留学生）的实验教学。

编者

2024 年 10 月

Preface

In 2019，the editor compiled and published the first edition of the national higher education pharmacy planning textbook *Experiments of Medicinal Chemistry*. This textbook has played an important role in teaching pharmacy major students，especially international students. In order to further meet the needs of the country and society for the cultivation of innovative pharmaceutical talents and the trend of internationalization of undergraduate teaching，we have revised the first edition of the textbook and compiled the bilingual textbook *Experiments of Medicinal Chemistry* (Second Edition).

Compared with the first edition of the textbook，this textbook retains the original 10 experiments and adds 9 new experiments，for a total of 19 experimental contents. The 9 newly added experiments are synthesis experiments of dipine drugs，peptide drugs，nucleoside drugs，and tinib drugs. In addition，this textbook also includes virtual simulation experiments on the synthesis of benzocaine (If you need to conduct virtual simulation experiments，please contact liwen@zzu. edu. cn)，enriching the structural categories，synthesis methods，and learning methods of drugs. The digital contents of experiments three to eight and twelve in this textbook is provided in the form of QR codes，mainly including demonstration videos of experimental operations. The newly added experiments not only include newly launched drugs in recent years，but also involve innovative drugs with independent intellectual property rights in China and the results of the editor's scientific research work.

This revision has added compound activity evaluation methods in the background knowledge section of each drug to deepen students' understanding of structure-activity relationships. In the experimental principle section of each drug，knowledge points have been added to help students understand and master the key learning points. In each drug synthesis experiment，a new method for determining drug content has been added to cultivate students' concept of drug quality. In the virtual simulation experiment of benzocaine synthesis，nuclear magnetic resonance hydrogen spectrum analysis of the compound was added to cultivate students' structural confirmation ability. The content of this textbook not only emphasizes the cultivation of students' ability in drug synthesis，but also fully reflects the comprehensiveness of knowledge such as drug design-chemical synthesis-structural confirmation-activity evaluation-content analysis. It is conducive to cultivating students' ability to flexibly apply pharmaceutical comprehensive knowledge and is a positive attempt to cultivate innovative talents.

Experiments 1 and 2 of this textbook were written by Wen Li and Yichao Zheng，experiments 7, 8, 9, and 14 were written by Wen Li, experiments 3 and 4 were written by Yajing Chen, experiment 5 was written by Lina Ding, experiment 6 was written by En Zhang, experiment 10 was written by Kai Sun, experiment 11 was written by Yingchao Duan, experiment 12 was written by Yichao Zheng, experiment 13 was written by Saiyang Zhang, experiment 15 was written by Peng Sang, experiment 16 was written by Yan Shi, experiment 17 was written by Yonggang Meng, experiment 18 was written by Xiaoyu Chang, experiment 19 was written by Xiaoyun Lu, and the entire book was reviewed by Qidong You. The part of the textbook on the mechanism of action of drug molecules and targets was prepared by Lina Ding and postgraduate students Ying Yan, Chaoya Ma, Zhizheng Wang, Qibing Gao, Xudong Sun, Jing Yang, Huan Liu, and Bingli Wang using MOE software for diagrams and writing. The section on drug activity evaluation methods in the textbook was written by Yichao Zheng. Muhammad Zeeshan, a doctoral student studying in China, and Linyuan Zhu, a graduate student, participated in the language editing work of this textbook.

This textbook is written in a bilingual system of Chinese and English, and can be used for experimental teaching of pharmacy majors (including international students) in higher medical colleges.

Editors
October 2024

前言（第一版）

为适应我国本科教学国际化的发展趋势，根据药物化学实验课程的基本要求，结合我们多年的教学经验和科研工作，编写了这本《药物化学实验双语教程（Experiments of Medicinal Chemistry）》。

本书包括 10 个化学药物合成实验，实验一至实验八为我们多年药物化学实验教学实践的总结，实验九和实验十为编者科研工作的结果。在化学药物合成实验的安排上，本书按照从基础操作到综合实验的顺序进行编写；在内容上，本书不仅给出了实验原理、操作过程、注意事项和思考题，而且给出了药物分子和靶标的作用机制图示、主要原料和中间体的物理常数、实验装置、安全提示和思考题参考答案。旨在强调药物化学理论教学与实验的关联，关注学生实验能力和科研素质培养。10 个化学药物合成实验的难易程度和实验学时有明显的区分度，可满足不同专业和不同层次学生的教学需求。

本教材的实验一、实验二、实验七、实验九由李雯、刘宏民编写，实验三、实验四由陈亚静编写，实验五由丁丽娜编写，实验六由张恩编写，实验八由郑一超编写，实验十由张秋荣编写，全书由尤启冬教授审订。书中药物分子和靶标的作用机制部分由丁丽娜及其研究生阎影、马超亚、王志正、高琦冰、孙旭东和杨晶等借助 MOE 软件进行模拟研究编写而成。留学中国的博士研究生 Moges Dessale Asmamaw、研究生常英杰、李瑞鹏及本科生朱林元参与了本书的语言润色工作。药物化学实验双语教材的建设，任重而道远。

《药物化学实验双语教程（Experiments of Medicinal Chemistry）》采用中英双语体系编写，可作为普通高等医药院校药学类各专业学生（包括留学生）的实验教材，也可供其他药学相关专业师生参考使用。

编者
2019 年 3 月

Preface (First Edition)

In order to adapt to the development trend of internationalization of undergraduate teaching in our country, according to the basic requirements of pharmaceutical chemistry experiment course combined with our years of teaching experience and scientific research work, this "bilingual course of pharmaceutical chemistry experiment" has been compiled.

In this textbook, 10 synthetic experiments of chemical drugs are included. Experiments 1 through 8 are the summaries of many years teaching practices, Experiments 9 and 10 are the results of the editors' scientific research work. They are arranged by the order from basic to comprehensive gradually. In each experiment, more than the experiment principle, operation process, notes and discussion questions are given, the action mechanism diagrams of drug molecule and target, physical constants of key raw materials and intermediates, experimental equipments, safety tips and reference answers of discussion questions are described. This textbook emphasizes the relationship between theoretical teaching and experiment of pharmaceutical chemistry, and pays attention to the cultivation of students' experimental ability and scientific research quality. There is a clear distinction between the difficulty and time of 10 experiments to meet the teaching needs of students from different majors and levels.

Experiments 1, 2, 7 and 9 of this textbook were written by Wen Li and Hongmin Liu, Experiments 3 and 4 by Yajing Chen, Experiment 5 by Lina Ding, Experiment 6 by En Zhang, Experiment 8 by Yichao Zheng and Experiment 10 by Qiurong Zhang. This textbook was revised by Professor Qidong You. The mechanistic studies between the drug molecule and the corresponding target were investigated and written by Lina Ding and her graduate students Ying Yan, Chaoya Ma, Zhizheng Wang, Qibing Gao, Xudong Sun and Jing Yang with the help of MOE software. We appreciate the foreign PhD student Moges Dessale Asmamaw, graduate students Yingjie Chang, Ruipeng Li and undergraduate student Linyuan Zhu who involved in the language correction of this textbook. The construction of bilingual textbooks is on the developing way.

This textbook is compiled in a Chinese-English bilingual system and can be used in the experimental teaching of pharmaceutical students (including foreign students) in medical colleges and universities.

Editors
March 2019

Contents
目　录

Experiment 1

Recrystallization of Acetanilide

Background

Acetanilide (Fig. 1-1) is an odourless solid chemical with a leaf or flake-like appearance. It is also known as N-phenylacetamide, acetanil, or acetanilid, and it was formerly known as the trade name Antifebrin.

Acetanilide is the first aniline derivative found to possess analgesic and antipyretic properties, and was quickly introduced into medical practice by A. Cahn and P. Hepp in 1886. But due to the unacceptable toxic effects, it was replaced by a new generation of acetyl drugs such as phenacetin and paracetamol (Fig. 1-1).

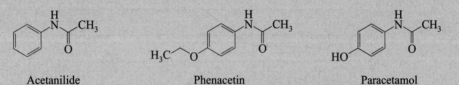

| Acetanilide | Phenacetin | Paracetamol |

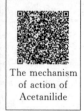

The mechanism of action of Acetanilide

Fig. 1-1   Chemical structures of Acetanilide, Phenacetin and Paracetamol

Now, acetanilide is mainly used as industrial rubber vulcanization promoter, stabilizer of fiber fat coating, stabilizer of hydrogen peroxide, and it also can be used for the synthesis of camphor.

I Purposes and Requirements

1. To master the recrystallization principle.
2. To master the operation of recrystallization.
3. To understand the interaction between acetanilide and target.

II Principle of the Reaction

1. Physical data of the main reactants and product

Name	Structure CAS No.	Formula M. Wt	b. p. or m. p. /℃	Solubility/(g/L)
Acetanilide	$\begin{array}{c}\text{H}\\\text{N}-\text{CH}_3\\\text{O}\end{array}$ 103-84-4	C_8H_9NO 135. 16	m. p. 113~115 b. p. 304	In water: 5. 5 (at 100 ℃) and 0. 46 (at 20 ℃) In ethanol: 36. 9 (at 20 ℃) In methanol: 69. 5 (at 20 ℃) In chloroform: 3. 6 (at 20 ℃)

2. Recrystallization principle

Compounds obtained from reaction mixtures always contain some impurities. The impurities may include some residues of soluble, insoluble and colored compounds. To obtain a pure product, these impurities must be completely removed.

Recrystallization is the primary method for purifying solid organic compounds. The principle of recrystallization is that the amount of solute that can be dissolved by a solvent increase with temperature. For example, the solubility curve of acetanilide in water with respect to varying temperature is shown in Fig. 1-2. The solubility of acetanilide increases from 4. 6 g/L to 55 g/L when the temperature increases from 20 ℃ to 100 ℃.

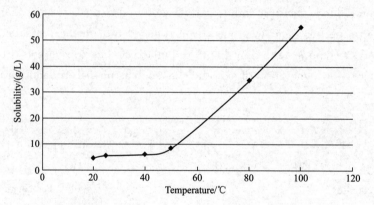

Fig. 1-2   Solubility curve of acetanilide in water

In a recrystallization procedure (Fig. 1-3), selection of an appropriate solvent is the most important factor. When an appropriate solvent is selected, solid compounds that contain some impurities can be dissolved in the solvent at or near their boiling points. The insoluble impurities can be removed by hot filtration. This step of recrystallization should be conducted while keeping the apparatus hot so as to

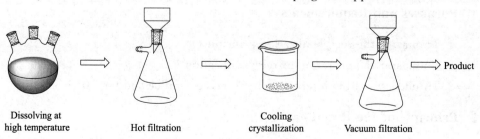

Dissolving at high temperature   Hot filtration   Cooling crystallization   Vacuum filtration   Product

Fig. 1-3   Procedure of recrystallization

prevent premature crystal formation. Next, allow the hot solution to cool down to room temperature before collecting the purified crystals by filtration. Note that the soluble impurities will remain in the filtrate.

The boiling points and dielectric constants of the commonly used solvents are summarized in Appendix 4.

3. Knowledge points

Difference in solubility of acetanilide at low and high temperatures.

Ⅲ Experimental Equipments and Raw Materials

1. Apparatus

The dissolving apparatus and the vacuum filtration apparatus

The dissolving apparatus is composed of a three-neck round-bottom flask, a spherical condenser tube, a magnetic stirrer and a thermometer.

The vacuum filtration apparatus is composed of a filter flask, a Buchner funnel, a filter paper and a vacuum pump.

2. Raw materials

Name	Quantity	Quality	Use
Acetanilide	2 g (0.015 mol)	Industrial grade	Raw material
Activated carbon (Charcoal)	0.5 g	—	Decolorizing substance
Distilled water	40 mL	—	Recrystallization solvent

Ⅳ Operations

(1) Equip the dissolving apparatus.

(2) Add 2 g of the impure acetanilide and 40 mL of distilled water into a 100 mL three-neck round-bottom flask.

(3) Dissolve the solute completely by stirring (magnetic stirrer) and heating the mixture to 100 ℃.

(4) Once acetanilide is dissolved completely, slightly cool down the solution to about 95 ℃ followed by the addition of 0.5 g of activated carbon. De-colorization is achieved by heating the mixture for about 10 minutes for gentle refluxing.

(5) Equip the vacuum filtration apparatus.

(6) Filter the hot solution by vacuum filtration. Allow the filtrate to cool down to room temperature in an ice-water bath for about 10 minutes. Caution should be taken not to shake or stir the filtrate.

(7) The pure product is collected by filtrating again. Attention should be paid to drain the solvent as far as possible.

(8) The product is dried under an infrared lamp. Weigh the pure product, calculate the yield and measure the melting point.

(9) Send the final product to the place where the teachers designated.

Ⅴ Experimental Results

1. Yield

Calculate the percent yield of acetanilide.

$$\text{Yield} = \frac{\text{Practical production}}{\text{Theoretical production}} \times 100\% = \frac{(\quad)}{2\text{ g}} \times 100\% = (\quad)\%$$

2. Appearance and melting point of the pure product

A. Appearance： _____ ;

B. m. p. ：

    Theoretical value：113～115 ℃ ；

    Practical value： _____ .

3. Analysis of experimental results

_____

_____

_____

_____

_____

_____

_____

_____

_____ .

Ⅵ Notes

1. In general, the amount of activated carbon is 1%～5% (by weight) of the crude product according to the color intensity.

2. Adding activated carbon while the solution is boiling can easily cause serious bumping. Therefore, when the activated carbon is added, the temperature of the solution must be slightly lower.

3. The filtrate of the hot solution should be allowed to cool slowly to room temperature. Gradual cooling is conducive for the formation of large well-defined crystals.

4. When the crystals are collected and washed, allow the water pump to run for several minutes so that the crystals have an opportunity to dry.

Ⅶ Determination of Product Content

The boiling point of acetanilide is 304℃, and gas chromatography (GC) can be used for content analysis.

Ⅷ Discussion Questions

1. Why the activated carbon can not be added to the boiling solution when it is used as a decolorizing agent?

2. What are the commonly used recrystallization solvents?

（By Wen Li, Yichao Zheng）

实验一

乙酰苯胺重结晶

> ### 背景知识
>
> 乙酰苯胺（Acetanilide）为无味、白色叶状或片状结晶（图1-1），也称作 N-苯基乙酰胺，曾以商品名退热冰应用于临床。
>
> 乙酰苯胺是第一个被发现的具有镇痛和解热作用的苯胺衍生物类化合物。1886年，A. Cahn 和 P. Hepp 将其应用于临床。但是，乙酰苯胺具有严重的副作用从而被新一代的乙酰苯胺类药物取代，比如非那西汀和对乙酰氨基酚。 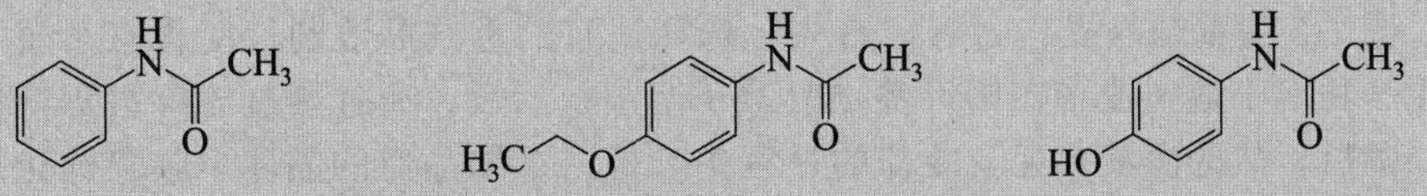
>
>
>
> 乙酰苯胺　　　　　　　　非那西汀　　　　　　　　对乙酰氨基酚
>
> 图1-1　乙酰苯胺、非那西汀和对乙酰氨基酚的化学结构
>
> 乙酰苯胺的作用机制
>
> 目前，乙酰苯胺主要用作工业橡胶硫化促进剂、纤维脂肪涂层稳定剂、双氧水稳定剂和合成樟脑。

Ⅰ 目的与要求

1. 掌握重结晶原理。
2. 掌握重结晶操作。
3. 了解乙酰苯胺与靶标的作用方式。

Ⅱ 实验原理

1. 主要反应物和产物的物理常数

名称	结构式 CAS号	分子式 分子量	沸点或熔点 /℃	溶解度/(g/L)
乙酰苯胺	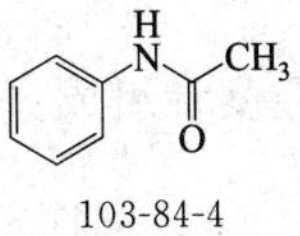 103-84-4	C_8H_9NO 135.16	m. p. 113~115 b. p. 304	水:55（100 ℃），4.6（20 ℃）； 乙醇:36.9（20 ℃）； 甲醇:69.5（20 ℃）； 氯仿:3.6（20 ℃）

2. 重结晶原理

反应获得的化合物往往含有一些杂质，这些杂质可以是可溶的、不易溶解的和有色的化合物。若要获得纯净的化合物，必须除去以上所述杂质。重结晶是除去固体化合物杂质的常用方法之一。

重结晶的原理是：一般情况下，溶质在溶液中的溶解度随着温度的升高而增大。例如，图 1-2 给出了乙酰苯胺在水中的溶解度曲线，在水中，当温度从 20 ℃升高到 100 ℃时，乙酰苯胺的溶解度从 4.6 g/L 增大至 55 g/L。

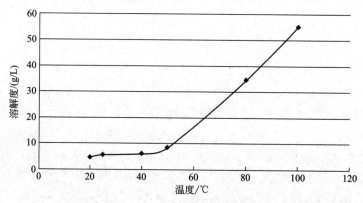

图 1-2　乙酰苯胺在水中的溶解度曲线

图 1-3 为重结晶操作过程。首先，选择适宜的重结晶溶剂，使含有杂质的固体化合物溶于溶剂或者在接近沸点时溶于溶剂；然后，通过热过滤除去不溶性杂质；随后，热的滤液在逐渐冷却的过程中，析出重结晶后的晶体，收集纯化后的产物，可溶性杂质留在滤液中。

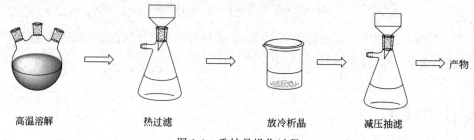

高温溶解　　　　　热过滤　　　　　放冷析晶　　　　减压抽滤

图 1-3　重结晶操作过程

重结晶溶剂的选取是非常重要的因素。常用的重结晶溶剂的沸点和介电常数汇总于附录四。

3. 知识点

乙酰苯胺在低温和高温时存在溶解度差异。

溶解和抽滤
装置

Ⅲ 实验装置和原料

1. 实验装置

溶解装置由三口烧瓶、回流冷凝管、磁力搅拌器和温度计组成。
抽滤装置由抽滤瓶、布氏漏斗、滤纸和真空泵组成。

2. 原料

名称	用量	试剂级别	用途
乙酰苯胺	2 g（0.015 mol）	工业级	原料
活性炭	0.5 g	—	脱色剂
蒸馏水	40 mL	—	重结晶溶剂

IV 实验操作

（1）搭建溶解装置。

（2）在 100 mL 三口烧瓶中，加入 2 g 乙酰苯胺粗品、40 mL 蒸馏水。

（3）边搅拌边升高温度至 100 ℃。

（4）溶解完全后，降温至 95 ℃，加入 0.5 g 活性炭。然后，加热至沸腾，并保持 10 min，脱色。

（5）搭建真空抽滤装置。

（6）热过滤，滤液静置放冷至室温，然后冰水浴 10 min，析出晶体。

（7）过滤沉淀，尽量抽干。

（8）产品干燥，称重，计算收率，测熔点。

（9）将产物送到指导教师指定的产品回收处。

V 实验结果

1. 收率

计算乙酰苯胺的收率。

$$收率 = \frac{产品实际产量}{产品理论产量} \times 100\% = \frac{(\quad\quad)}{2\ g} \times 100\% = (\quad\quad)\%$$

2. 产品外观与熔点

A. 外观：_____；

B. 熔点：

理论值：113～115 ℃；

实测值：_____。

3. 实验结果分析

_____

_____

_____

_____

_____

_____

_____。

VI 注意事项

1. 一般情况下，根据粗品颜色的深浅程度，活性炭的用量为粗品质量的 1%～5%。

2. 当溶液沸腾时，加入活性炭易引起暴沸。因此，加入活性炭时，需要将溶液稍微降降温。

3. 经热过滤获得的滤液，在降温至室温的过程中，需要缓慢降温。缓慢降温是获得较大粒度、完好晶体的关键因素。

4. 当晶体过滤和洗涤后，应让真空泵继续抽气几分钟，以使得获得的晶体尽可能干燥。

Ⅶ 产物的含量测定

乙酰苯胺的沸点为 304℃，可采用气相色谱法（gas chromatography，GC）进行含量分析。

Ⅷ 思考题

1. 活性炭脱色时，为什么不能将活性炭加入到沸腾的溶液中？
2. 常用的重结晶溶剂有哪些？

（李雯　郑一超）

Experiment 2

Synthesis of Aspirin

Background

Salicylic acid was isolated from the willow bark tree and the chemical structure was defined in 1823 (Fig. 2-1). Since then, salicylic acid is widely used in the clinical practice as anti-rheumatic and antipyretic analgesic drug. However, it has apparent stomach-stimulating effects that can induce gastrointestinal discomfort and peptic ulcer disease among others.

Aspirin is derived from salicylic acid by substituting the phenolic hydroxy group on benzene cycle with the acetoxyl group (Fig. 2-1). Due to this aspirin has a much lower side effect than salicylic acid. In addition, the modification also extends the clinical use of aspirin to anti-thrombosis, which exhibits beneficial effects in the prevention and treatment of cardiovascular diseases, such as coronary heart disease and atherosclerosis.

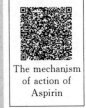
The mechanism of action of Aspirin

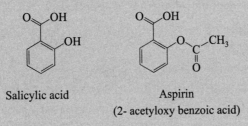

Salicylic acid

Aspirin
(2- acetyloxy benzoic acid)

Fig. 2-1　Chemical structure of Salicylic acid and Aspirin

I Purposes and Requirements

1. To master the acetylation reaction and its use in structural modification of drug substances.

2. To master the anhydrous operation method, and the use of coloration reaction on the endpoint detection of organic synthesis.

3. To understand the interaction between aspirin and target.

Ⅱ Principle of the Reaction

1. Physical data of the main reactants and product

Name	Structure CAS No.	Formula M. Wt	b. p. or m. p. /℃	Solubility
Salicylic acid	(structure) 69-72-7	$C_7H_6O_3$ 138. 12	m. p. 158~161	In water: 1. 8 g/L (at 20 ℃) In ethanol: 1 mol/L (at 20 ℃)
Acetic anhydride	(structure) 108-24-7	$C_4H_6O_3$ 102. 09	b. p. 138~139	Reaction with water to form acetic acid; and miscible with ether, chloroform and benzene
Aspirin	(structure) 50-78-2	$C_9H_8O_4$ 180. 16	m. p. 135~138	In water: 3. 3 g/L (at 20 ℃) In DMSO: 100 mmol/L (at 20 ℃)

2. Synthetic Route

Salicylic acid + Acetic anhydride $\xrightarrow{H_2SO_4}$ Aspirin + Acetic acid

Aspirin is synthesized by an acylation reaction using salicylic acid and acetic anhydride as starting materials. The reaction is catalyzed by concentrated sulfuric acid and should take place in an anhydrous environment.

The reaction for endpoint detection is as follows:

$$3 \text{(structure)} + FeCl_3 \longrightarrow Fe^{3+}\text{(structure)}_3 + 3 HCl$$

Light red color

Safety Tips: The acetic anhydride and sulfuric acid can cause bad burns and thus will be used in the hood. If they come in contact with your skin, immediately wash the area with copious amounts of water.

3. Knowledge points

Acylation reaction, acetic anhydride serves as the acylation reagent, reaction endpoint detection.

Ⅲ Experimental Equipments and Raw Materials

1. Experimental equipments

The reaction apparatus is composed of a three-neck round-bottom flask , a

Reaction apparatus of synthesis of Aspirin

spherical condenser tube, a magnetic stirrer and a thermometer.

2. Raw materials

Name	Quantity	Quality	Use
Salicyclic acid	8.3 g (0.06 mol)	CP	Reactant
Acetic anhydride	15 mL (0.159 mol)	CP	Acetylating agent
Sulfuric acid	0.4 mL (5 drops)	CP	Catalyst
$FeCl_3$ reagent	1 drop	—	Endpoint indicator
Ethanol	12 mL	95%	Solvent for recryst
H_2O	Proper amount	—	Solvent
Active carbon (Charcoal)	0.5 g	—	Decolorizing substance

Ⅳ Operations

1. Synthesis of aspirin crude product

(1) Equip the reaction apparatus.

(2) Add 15 mL of acetic anhydride and 5 drops of concentrated sulfuric acid into a 100 mL three-neck round-bottom flask. Heat the solution to 55~60 ℃ while stirring with a magnetic stirrer.

Experimental procedure of synthesis of aspirin crude product

(3) Keep the solution at 55~60 ℃ and add 8.3 g of salicylic acid to the reaction flask. The white crystals can be observed to dissolve gradually with stirring.

(4) Endpoint detection. One drop of reaction solution is taken out and put into the reaction board. The reaction solution should be changed to yellow upon the addition of one drop of $FeCl_3$ reagent. The reaction solution should not show violet. If the solution shows light violet, then the reaction needs to be continued.

(5) If the reaction reaches the endpoint, cool the flask to room temperature and then put it into a cold water-bath. Add 75 mL of water to the flask and collect the product by vacuum filtration.

(6) Wash the product 2~3 times with ice water. Attention should be paid to drain the solvent as far as possible.

(7) Dry the product under an infrared lamp and measure the weight.

2. Recrystallization of aspirin

(1) Equip the reaction apparatus.

(2) Add the crude product (aspirin) and 12 mL ethanol into a 100 mL three-neck round-bottom flask. Dissolve the solute completely by stirring (magnetic stirrer) and heating the mixture to 50 ℃.

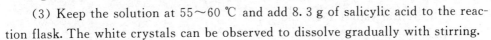
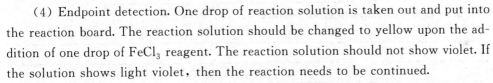

Experiment procedure of recrystallization of aspirin

(3) Once the crude product (aspirin) is dissolved completely, 0.5 g of activated carbon (decolorizing substance) is added to the reaction mixture at 50 ℃. Then, the mixture is kept at 50 ℃ for 5 minutes to decolorize the product.

(4) Filter the hot solution by vacuum filtration. Allow the filtrate to cool down to room temperature (just put the filtrate on the experiment table). Add 12 mL of cold distilled water to the filtrate and collect the pure product by filtering again.

(5) Wash the pure product 2~3 times with 30% ethanol. Attention should be paid to drain the solvent as far as possible.

(6) The product is dried under an infrared lamp. Weigh the pure product, calculate the yield and measure the melting point.

(7) Send the final product to the place where the teachers designated.

Ⅴ Experimental Results

1. Yield

(1) Calculate the theoretical production of aspirin

$$\text{Salicyclic acid} \longrightarrow \text{Aspirin}$$
$$M_w = 138.12 \text{ g/mol} \longrightarrow M_w = 180.16 \text{ g/mol}$$
$$0.06 \text{ mol} \longrightarrow 0.06 \text{ mol}$$

Theoretical production = 0.06 mol × 180.16 g/mol = 10.81 g

(2) Calculate the percent yield of aspirin

$$\text{Yield} = \frac{\text{Practical production}}{\text{Theoretical production}} \times 100\% = \frac{(\quad)}{10.81 \text{ g}} \times 100\% = (\quad)\%$$

2. Appearance and melting point of product

A. Appearance: _____ ;

B. m. p. :

Theoretical value: 135~138 ℃ ;

Practical value: _____ .

3. Analysis of experimental results

_____

_____

_____

_____

_____

_____

_____

_____

_____ .

Ⅵ Notes

1. During the synthesis of the crude product, the anhydrous condition is the first decisive factor. The reason is that acetic anhydride can be decomposed by moist air or water. So, all apparatus and raw materials should be absolutely dried.

2. Controlling the reaction temperature is the second decisive factor. This is due to the fact that when the reaction temperature is above 60 ℃, salicylic acid will be oxidized by H_2SO_4 (a strong oxidizing agent) and it will change into a yellow or dark oxidized product. So, the reaction and the recrystallization temperature must be controlled below 60 ℃.

Ⅶ Determination of Product Content

Acid-base titration method: Take about 0.4g of this product, weigh it accurately, dissolve it in 20 mL of neutral ethanol (neutral to phenolphthalein indicator solution), add 3 drops of phenolphthalein indicator solution, and titrate with sodium hydroxide titrant (0.1 mol/L). Every 1 mL of sodium hydroxide titrant (0.1 mol/L) is equivalent to 18.02 mg of aspirin. (《Chinese Pharmacopoeia》 2020 Edition)

Ⅷ Discussion Questions

1. In terms of structure, why dose/might our room smell like vinegar during this experiment?

2. In terms of structure, why are salicylic and acetylsalicylic acid considered as acids?

(By Wen Li, Yichao Zheng)

阿司匹林的合成

背景知识

1823 年，药物化学家从柳树皮中分离获得了水杨酸，并确证了其化学结构（图 2-1）。此后，水杨酸作为抗风湿和解热镇痛药物被广泛应用。然而，水杨酸具有明显的胃刺激作用，可引起胃不适症状和消化性溃疡等副作用。

当把水杨酸的酚羟基酰化为乙酰氧基，便得到了阿司匹林（图 2-1）。阿司匹林的副作用远低于水杨酸。此外，阿司匹林的临床应用还扩展至抗血栓治疗，对冠心病、动脉粥样硬化等心血管疾病的防治也有积极作用。

水杨酸

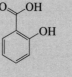

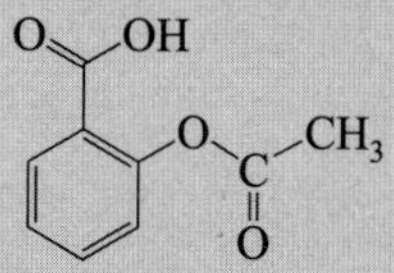

阿司匹林
(2-乙酰氧基水杨酸)

图 2-1　水杨酸和阿司匹林的化学结构

（左侧边栏）阿司匹林的作用机制

Ⅰ　目的与要求

1. 掌握酯化反应原理和其在药物结构改造中的应用。
2. 掌握无水反应操作，掌握颜色反应在反应终点判断方面的应用。
3. 了解阿司匹林与靶标的作用方式。

Ⅱ　实验原理

1. 主要反应物和产物的物理常数

名称	结构式 CAS 号	分子式 分子量	沸点或熔点/℃	溶解度
水杨酸	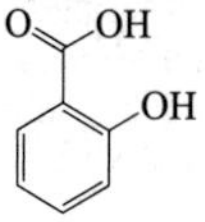 69-72-7	$C_7H_6O_3$ 138.12	m. p. 158～161	水：1.8 g/L（20 ℃）；乙醇：1 mol/L（20 ℃）

名称	结构式 CAS 号	分子式 分子量	沸点或熔点/℃	溶解度
乙酸酐	H_3C—C(=O)—O—C(=O)—CH_3 108-24-7	$C_4H_6O_3$ 102.09	b. p. 138～139	遇水反应,生成醋酸;易溶于乙醚、氯仿和苯
阿司匹林	COOH—O—C(=O)—CH_3(苯环) 50-78-2	$C_9H_8O_4$ 180.16	m. p. 135～138	水:3.3 g/L(20 ℃); DMSO:100 mmol/L(20 ℃)

2. 合成路线

水杨酸 + 乙酸酐 $\xrightarrow{H_2SO_4}$ 阿司匹林 + CH_3COOH

水杨酸　　　　　　乙酸酐　　　　　　　　阿司匹林　　　　　醋酸

水杨酸与乙酸酐在浓硫酸催化下,发生酰化反应生成阿司匹林和醋酸。反应在无水条件下进行,所有试剂和反应仪器应在反应前干燥,并在反应过程中严格避水。

反应终点检测的反应式如下:

$$3 \text{(水杨酸)} + FeCl_3 \longrightarrow Fe^{3+}\left(\text{(水杨酸根)}\right)_3 + 3\ HCl$$

淡红色

安全提示:乙酸酐和浓硫酸会引起严重烧伤。使用时应戴上手套,如果接触皮肤,立即用大量水冲洗。

3. 知识点

乙酰化反应,乙酸酐为酰化试剂,反应终点检测。

Ⅲ 实验装置和原料

1. 实验装置

反应装置由三口烧瓶、回流冷凝管、磁力搅拌器和温度计组成。

阿司匹林合成反应装置

2. 原料

名称	用量	试剂级别	用途
水杨酸	8.3 g(0.06 mol)	化学纯	反应物
乙酸酐	15 mL(0.159 mol)	化学纯	酰化试剂
浓硫酸	0.4 mL(5 滴)	化学纯	催化剂
$FeCl_3$ 试液	1 滴	—	终点指示剂

名称	用量	试剂级别	用途
乙醇	12 mL	95%	重结晶溶剂
H_2O	适量	—	溶剂
活性炭	0.5 g	—	脱色剂

Ⅳ 实验操作

1. 阿司匹林粗品合成

（1）搭建反应装置。

（2）在 100 mL 三口烧瓶中，加入 15 mL 乙酸酐和 5 滴浓硫酸，搅拌状态下，升温至 55～60 ℃。

（3）在以上体系中，加入 8.3 g 水杨酸晶体，55～60 ℃ 下搅拌溶解，可观察到白色晶体逐渐溶解。

（4）终点检测：取一滴反应液，滴到反应板上，再滴入一滴 $FeCl_3$ 试剂，反应液不可以显示粉红色（必须显示黄色），若反应液显示淡红色，反应需要继续。

（5）若反应达到终点，停止反应，使反应液冷却至室温，把反应瓶放入冰水浴，加入 75 mL 水，减压抽滤，收集产品。

（6）冰水洗涤产品 2～3 次，尽量抽干。

（7）风干粗品，称重。

2. 粗品纯化

（1）搭建反应装置。

（2）在 100 mL 三口烧瓶中，将阿司匹林粗品溶于 12 mL 乙醇中，升高温度至 50 ℃。

（3）粗品完全溶解后，加入 0.5 g 活性炭，50 ℃ 下保持 5 min 以脱色。

（4）热过滤，将滤液置于实验台，冷却，加入 12 mL 冰水，再次过滤，获得阿司匹林纯品。

（5）用 30% 乙醇洗涤纯品 2～3 次，尽量抽干。

（6）风干纯品，称重，计算收率，测熔点。

（7）将产物送到指导教师指定的产品回收处。

Ⅴ 实验结果

1. 收率

（1）计算阿司匹林的理论产量。

$$水杨酸 \longrightarrow 阿司匹林$$
$$M_w = 138.12 \text{ g/mol} \longrightarrow M_w = 180.16 \text{ g/mol}$$
$$0.06 \text{ mol} \longrightarrow 0.06 \text{ mol}$$
$$理论产量 = 0.06 \text{ mol} \times 180.16 \text{ g/mol} = 10.81 \text{ g}$$

（2）计算阿司匹林的收率

$$收率 = \frac{产品实际产量}{产品理论产量} \times 100\% = \frac{(\quad)}{10.81 \text{ g}} \times 100\% = (\quad)\%$$

2. 产品外观与熔点

    A. 外观：_____；

    B. 熔点：

        理论值：135～138 ℃；

        实测值：_____。

3. 实验结果分析

_____

_____

_____

_____

_____

_____

_____。

Ⅵ 注意事项

1. 粗品制备过程中，无水条件是至关重要的因素。这是因为乙酸酐在水中或湿空气中会发生分解，因此，该步反应需要在完全无水条件下完成。

2. 粗品制备过程中，反应温度控制是第二个重要的因素。这是因为浓硫酸是强氧化剂，当反应温度为 60 ℃以上时，水杨酸会被浓硫酸氧化为黄色或棕黑色产物，因此，反应和重结晶温度必须控制在 60 ℃以下。

Ⅶ 产物的含量测定

酸碱滴定法：取本品约 0.4 g，精密称定，加中性乙醇（对酚酞指示液显中性）20 mL 溶解后，加酚酞指示液 3 滴，用氢氧化钠滴定液（0.1 mol/L）滴定。每 1 mL 氢氧化钠滴定液（0.1 mol/L）相当于 18.02 mg 的阿司匹林。（《中华人民共和国药典（2020 年版）》）

Ⅷ 思考题

1. 用结构式表示，为什么反应过程中室内会有醋酸的味道？

2. 用结构式表示，为什么水杨酸和阿司匹林是酸性物质？

（李雯　郑一超）

Experiment 3

Synthesis of Paracetamol

Background

Paracetamol (APAP), also known as acetaminophen, is a non-antiinflammatory antipyretic analgesic drug of anilines. It has a similar antipyretic effect with aspirin but weaker analgesic effect and neither anti-inflammatory nor anti-rheumatism effect.

APAP is clinically used in the treatment of fever, headache, arthralgia, neuralgia, etc. Paracetamol is also the active constituent of anti-influenza compounds, such as Quike capsule for the treatment of the common cold. The chemical structure of paracetamol is shown in Fig. 3-1.

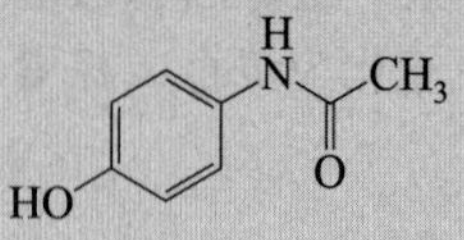

Fig. 3-1　Chemical structure of Paracetamol

The mechanism of action of Paracetamol

I　Purposes and Requirements

1. To master the principle and operation techniques of acylation reaction.
2. To master the recrystallization method.
3. To know well the use of antioxidants and the protection of medicine from oxidation.
4. To understand the interaction between paracetamol and target.

II　Principle of the Reaction

1. Physical data of the main reactants and product

Name	Structure CAS No.	Formula M. Wt	b. p. or m. p. /℃	Solubility
Para-aminophenol	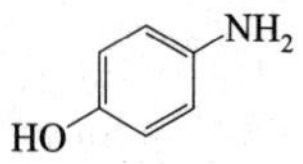 123-30-8	C_6H_7NO 109. 13	m. p. 188~190	1. 5 g/100 mL (at 20 ℃) in water, miscible with organic solvent

Name	Structure CAS No.	Formula M. Wt	b. p. or m. p. /℃	Solubility
Acetic anhydride	H₃C–CO–O–CO–CH₃ 108-24-7	$C_4H_6O_3$ 102. 09	b. p. 138~139	React with water to form acetic acid and miscible with ether, chloroform and benzene
Paracetamol	HO–C₆H₄–NH–CO–CH₃ 103-90-2	$C_8H_9NO_2$ 151. 16	m. p. 168~172	1. 4 g/100 mL（at 20 ℃）in water, miscible with organic solvent
Sodium hydrogen sulfite	NaHSO₃ 7631-90-5	$NaHSO_3$ 104. 06	m. p. 150~152	Soluble in water and slightly soluble in ethanol

2. Synthetic route

Para-aminophenol   Acetic anhydride   Paracetamol   Acetic acid

In this reaction，*Para*-aminophenol will react with acetic anhydride to form paracetamol and one molecule of acetic acid.

Safety Tips：Acetic anhydride can cause bad burns and thus should always be used in the hood. If it comes in contact with your skin，immediately wash the area with copious amounts of water.

3. Knowledge points

Acylation reaction，recrystallization，antioxidant.

Ⅲ Experimental Equipments and Raw Materials

1. Experimental equipments

The reaction apparatus，is composed of a three-neck round-bottom flask，a spherical condenser tube，a magnetic stirrer and a thermometer.

The purification apparatus is composed of a beaker，a magnetic stirrer，and a thermometer.

Reaction apparatus of synthesis of Paracetamol

2. Raw materials

Name	Quantity	Quality	Use
Para-aminophenol	10. 6 g（0. 097 mol）	CP	Reactant
Acetic anhydride	12 mL（0. 127 mol）	CP	Acylation agent
Water	30 mL	—	Solvent
Active carbon (Charcoal)	1 g	—	Decolorization
NaHSO₃	0. 5 g（0. 005 mol）	CP	Antioxidant

Ⅳ Operations

1. Synthesis and isolation (for obtaining the crude product)

（1）Equip the dissolving apparatus.

（2）Add 10. 6 g of *para*-aminophenol，30 mL of water and 12 mL of acetic anhydride to a 100 mL three-neck round-bottom flask and agitate gently in parallel. Heat the solution to 80 ℃ on a steam bath for 30 minutes，and then cool it by putting it in ice-water bath for 20 minutes to crystallize out. （We can use a glass rod to rub the beaker to increases the rate of cry stallization. ）

（3）Filter it and collect the crystals，wash them with 10 mL of cold water twice and dry the crystals of the obtained crude product.

2. Recrystallization (for purification)

（1）Equip the dissolving apparatus.

（2）Weigh the crude product. Place it in a 250 mL beaker and dissolve it in an adequate amount of water（the ratio is 5 mL water for 1 g of the product），and then，agitate gently in parallel.

（3）Raise the temperature to 85 ℃ to dissolve. The mixture is cooled down to 75 ℃ after dissolving. Add 1 g of active carbon to the mixture. Then，increase the temperature to 100 ℃ for boiling and keep for 5 minutes to decolor.

（4）Filter the hot reaction solution（before filtering，add 0. 5 g of $NaHSO_3$ into preheated filter flash to avoid oxidation of the product）. The filtrate is cooled to crystallize out.

（5）Filter the mixture. Wash the filter cake twice with 5 mL of 0. 5％ $NaHSO_3$ solution.

（6）Dry the product under an infrared light to obtain a white solid. Weigh the pure product and measure the melting point.

（7）Send the product to the place where the teachers designated.

Ⅴ Experimental Results

1. Yield

（1）Calculate the theoretical production of paracetamol

$$Para\text{-aminophenol} \longrightarrow \text{Paracetamol}$$
$$M_w = 109. 13 \text{ g/mol} \longrightarrow M_w = 151. 16 \text{ g/mol}$$
$$0. 097 \text{ mol} \longrightarrow 0. 097 \text{ mol}$$

Theoretical production＝0. 097 mol×151. 16 g/mol＝14. 66 g

（2）Calculate the percent yield of paracetamol

$$\text{Yield} = \frac{\text{Practical production}}{\text{Theoretical production}} \times 100\% = \frac{(\quad)}{14. 66 \text{ g}} \times 100\% = (\quad)\%$$

2. Appearance and melting point of product

A. Appearance：_____ ；

B. m. p. ：

Theoretical value：169～171 ℃；

Practical value: _____.

3. Analysis of experimental results

_____

_____

_____

_____

_____

_____.

Ⅵ Notes

1. The purpose of adding sodium hydrogen sulfite is to avoid the oxidation of paracetamol by air. However, the concentration of sodium hydrogen sulfite should be under proper control, otherwise, the product's quality will be affected.

2. When performing hot filtration, the filter bottle and Buchner funnel need to be preheated in advance, and the filtration should be completed as soon as possible.

Ⅶ Determination of Product Content

Measure by UV visible spectrophotometry (General Rule 0401).

Measurement method: Take the test solution and measure the absorbance at a wavelength of 257 nm. Calculate based on the absorption coefficient ($E_{1cm}^{1\%}$) of acetaminophen, which is 715. (《Chinese Pharmacopoeia》 2020 Edition)

Ⅷ Discussion Questions

1. Can acetic acid be used as an acylating agent in this preparation?
2. What are the common acylating agents?
3. What are the common impurities of paracetamol?

(By Yajing Chen)

实验三

对乙酰氨基酚的合成

背景知识

对乙酰氨基酚（扑热息痛）是一种苯胺类非抗炎解热镇痛药，其解热作用类似于阿司匹林，但镇痛作用较弱，且不具有抗炎和抗风湿作用。对乙酰氨基酚临床上用于治疗发热，头痛、关节痛和神经痛等。对乙酰氨基酚是多种抗感冒复方制剂的活性成分，比如快克胶囊。对乙酰氨基酚的化学结构如图 3-1 所示。

图 3-1　对乙酰氨基酚的化学结构

对乙酰氨基酚的作用机制

Ⅰ　目的与要求

1. 熟悉和掌握乙酰化反应的原理和实验方法。
2. 掌握重结晶法进行纯化的实验方法。
3. 熟悉抗氧剂的使用及易氧化药物的保护。
4. 了解对乙酰氨基酚与靶标的作用方式。

Ⅱ　反应原理

1. 主要反应物及产物的物理常数

名称	结构式 CAS 号	分子式 分子量	沸点或 熔点/℃	溶解度
对氨基苯酚	123-30-8	C_6H_7NO 109.13	m. p. 188～190	1.5 g/100 mL（20 ℃）（水），易溶于常用有机溶剂
乙酸酐	108-24-7	$C_4H_6O_3$ 102.09	b. p. 138～139	遇水反应，生成醋酸；易溶于乙醚，氯仿和苯

22　药物化学实验（双语）（Experiments of Medicinal Chemistry）（第二版）

名称	结构式 CAS 号	分子式 分子量	沸点或 熔点/℃	溶解度
对乙酰氨基酚	HO—⟨⟩—N(H)—C(O)—CH₃ 103-90-2	$C_8H_9NO_2$ 151.16	m.p. 168～172	1.4 g/100 mL（20 ℃）（水），易溶于常用有机溶剂
亚硫酸氢钠	$NaHSO_3$ 7631-90-5	$NaHSO_3$ 104.06	m.p. 150～152	易溶于水，微溶于乙醇

2. 合成路线

$$HO-\langle\rangle-NH_2 \; + \; H_3C-C(O)-O-C(O)-CH_3 \quad \xrightarrow[80℃,\,30\ min]{H_2O} \quad HO-\langle\rangle-N(H)-C(O)-CH_3 \; + \; H_3C-C(O)-OH$$

对氨基苯酚　　　　　乙酸酐　　　　　　　　　　　　　对乙酰氨基酚　　　　乙酸

在此反应过程中，对氨基苯酚和乙酸酐反应生成对乙酰氨基酚，同时也会产生一分子乙酸。

安全提示：乙酸酐可灼伤皮肤，并有刺激性味道，应在通风橱中使用。一旦接触皮肤，要立即用大量水冲洗。

3. 知识点

酰化反应，重结晶，抗氧剂。

Ⅲ 实验装置和原料

1. 实验装置

乙酰化反应装置由三口烧瓶、回流冷凝管、磁力搅拌器和温度计组成。
精制反应装置由烧杯、磁力搅拌器和温度计组成。

乙酰化反应
装置和精制
反应装置

2. 原料

名称	用量	规格	用途
对氨基苯酚	10.6 g（0.097 mol）	化学纯	反应物
乙酸酐	12 mL（0.127 mol）	化学纯	乙酰化试剂
水	30 mL	—	溶剂
活性炭	1 g	—	脱色
亚硫酸氢钠	0.5 g（0.005 mol）	化学纯	抗氧剂

Ⅳ 实验操作

1. 对乙酰氨基酚的制备（粗品）

（1）搭建反应实验装置。

（2）于干燥的 100 mL 三口烧瓶中加入 10.6 g 对氨基苯酚、30 mL 水和 12 mL 乙酸酐，轻轻振摇使成均相。于 80 ℃ 蒸汽浴中加热反应 30 min，冰水浴中冷却 20 min，析晶。

（3）抽滤，滤饼用 10 mL 冷水洗 2 次，干燥，称重。

2. 重结晶（精制）

（1）搭建反应实验装置。

（2）于 250 mL 烧杯中，加入对乙酰氨基酚粗品，每克粗品用水 5 mL，加入计算量的水。

（3）加热至 85 ℃使其溶解，溶解后稍冷至 75 ℃，加入 1 g 活性炭，重新加热至 100 ℃，煮沸 5 min。

（4）趁热抽滤（抽滤前，将布氏漏斗和抽滤瓶在 80 ℃烘箱中预热 30 min，并在预热后的抽滤瓶中先加入 0.5 g 亚硫酸氢钠），滤液冷却析晶。

（5）抽滤。滤饼以 0.5％亚硫酸氢钠溶液 5 mL 分 2 次洗涤。

（6）红外灯下烘干产品，得白色固体。称重，计算收率，测熔点。

（7）将产物送到指导教师指定的产品回收处。

Ⅴ 实验结果

1. 收率

（1）计算对乙酰氨基酚的理论产量

$$对氨基苯酚 \text{————} 对乙酰氨基酚$$
$$M_w = 109.13 \text{ g/mol} \text{————} M_w = 151.16 \text{ g/mol}$$
$$0.097 \text{ mol} \text{————} 0.097 \text{ mol}$$
$$理论产量 = 0.097 \text{ mol} \times 151.16 \text{ g/mol} = 14.66 \text{ g}$$

（2）计算对乙酰氨基酚的收率

$$收率 = \frac{产品实际产量}{产品理论产量} \times 100\% = \frac{(\qquad)}{14.66 \text{ g}} \times 100\% = (\qquad)\%$$

2. 产品外观与熔点

A. 外观：＿＿＿＿＿＿＿＿＿＿＿＿＿＿＿＿＿＿＿＿；

B. 熔点：

理论值：169～171 ℃

实测值：＿＿＿＿＿＿＿＿＿＿＿＿＿＿＿＿。

3. 实验结果分析

＿＿＿＿＿＿＿＿＿＿＿＿＿＿＿＿＿＿＿＿＿＿＿＿＿＿＿＿＿＿＿＿＿＿＿＿

＿＿＿＿＿＿＿＿＿＿＿＿＿＿＿＿＿＿＿＿＿＿＿＿＿＿＿＿＿＿＿＿＿＿＿＿

＿＿＿＿＿＿＿＿＿＿＿＿＿＿＿＿＿＿＿＿＿＿＿＿＿＿＿＿＿＿＿＿＿＿＿＿

＿＿＿＿＿＿＿＿＿＿＿＿＿＿＿＿＿＿＿＿＿＿＿＿＿＿＿＿＿＿＿＿＿＿＿＿

＿＿＿＿＿＿＿＿＿＿＿＿＿＿＿＿＿＿＿＿＿＿＿＿＿＿＿＿＿＿＿＿＿＿＿＿

＿＿＿＿＿＿＿＿＿＿＿＿＿＿＿＿＿＿＿＿＿＿＿＿＿＿＿＿＿＿＿＿＿＿。

Ⅵ 注意事项

1. 加亚硫酸氢钠可防止对乙酰氨基酚被空气氧化，但亚硫酸氢钠浓度不宜过高，否则会影响产品质量。

2. 进行热过滤时，抽滤瓶和布氏漏斗需要提前预热，抽滤应尽快完成操作。

Ⅶ 产物的含量测定

照紫外-可见分光光度法（通则 0401）测定。

测定法：取供试品溶液，在 257 nm 的波长处测定吸光度，按对乙酰氨基酚的吸收系数（$E_{1cm}^{1\%}$）为 715 计算。（《中华人民共和国药典（2020 年版）》）

Ⅷ 思考题

1. 本实验中乙酸可以作为乙酰化试剂来使用吗？
2. 常用的乙酰化试剂有哪些？
3. 合成对乙酰氨基酚时常见的杂质有哪些？

（陈亚静）

Experiment 4
Synthesis of Benorilate

Background

Benorilate is a prodrug formed by the combination of aspirin and paraceta-mol. Clinically, it is used for the treatment of rheumatoid arthritis, cold-fervescence, neuralgia, and others. The therapeutic effect of benorilate is similar to that of aspirin but with a longer duration of action and fewer side effects. The chemical structure of benorilate is as follow Fig. 4-1.

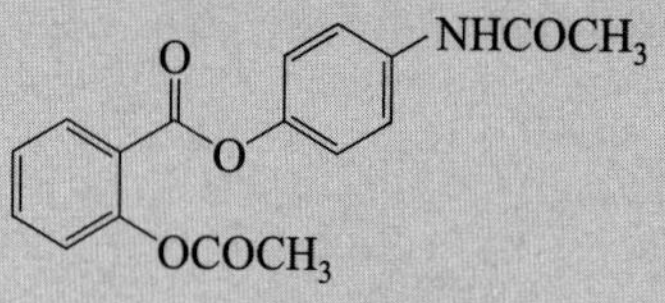

Fig. 4-1　Chemical structure of Benorilate

I　Purposes and Requirements

1. To understand the principle of chlorization and its requirements.

2. To understand the application of the combination principle in chemical structure modification.

3. To learn the treatment method of toxic gas produced during the reaction.

4. To master the technique of anhydrous operation of the reaction.

5. To understand the principle of Schotten-Baumann esterification.

6. To understand the interaction between benorilate and target.

II　Principle of the Reaction

1. Physical data of the main reactants and product

Name	Structure CAS No.	Formula M. Wt	b. p. or m. p. /℃	Solubility
Aspirin	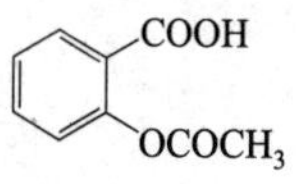 COOH OCOCH$_3$ 50-78-2	C$_9$H$_8$O$_4$ 180. 16	m. p. 135～138	In water: 3. 3 g/L (at 20 ℃) In DMSO: 100 mmol/L (at 20 ℃)

Name	Structure CAS No.	Formula M. Wt	b. p. or m. p. /℃	Solubility
2-(Acetyloxy)-benzoylchlorid	COCl / OCOCH₃ 5538-51-2	$C_9H_7O_3Cl$ 198. 60	m. p. 45~49	Soluble in toluene Decomposed in water
Thionyl chloride	$SOCl_2$ 7719-09-7	$SOCl_2$ 118. 97	b. p. 79	React with water and miscible with organic solvents
Pyridine	N 110-86-1	C_5H_5N 79. 10	b. p. 115	Soluble in water and common organic solvents
Paracetamol	HO—N(H)—COCH₃ 103-90-2	$C_8H_9NO_2$ 151. 16	m. p. 168~172	In water: 1. 4 g/100 mL (at 20 ℃) Miscible in organic solvent In ethanol: 0.5 mol/L (at 20 ℃)
Benorilate	NHCOCH₃ / O / OCOCH₃ 5003-48-5	$C_{17}H_{15}NO_5$ 313. 31	m. p. 177~181	Insoluble in water Easily soluble in hot ethanol

2. Synthetic route

(1)

$$\text{COOH / OCOCH}_3 + SOCl_2 \xrightarrow{\text{N}} \text{COCl / OCOCH}_3 + HCl + SO_2$$

(2)

$$\text{HO—N(H)—COCH}_3 + NaOH \longrightarrow \text{NaO—N(H)—COCH}_3 + H_2O$$

(3)

$$\text{COCl / OCOCH}_3 + \text{NaO—N(H)—COCH}_3 \longrightarrow \text{NHCOCH}_3 \text{ ester / OCOCH}_3 + NaCl$$

During Benorilate synthesis, the phenol group of paracetamol reacts with the carboxyl group of aspirin to form an ester product. Aspirin is an aromatic acid which has low reactivity. In this experiment, aspirin is first treated with thionyl chloride and pyridine to form the corresponding acetyl salicylic chloride under an anhydrous reaction condition. Considering the similar low reactivity of the phenol group of the paracetamol, paracetamol is changed to its sodium salt in a sodium hydroxide solution. Finally, the two intermediates formed then react at room temperature to form benorilate.

Safety Tips: Thionyl chloride and pyridine have an irritating smell and thus should be used in the hood. If treated otherwise, they can burn the skin, irritate the mucous membrane. Thionyl chloride and the produced acetyl salicylic chloride can react violently with water and liberate toxic gas.

3. Knowledge points

Chlorination reaction, absorption of acidic gases, principle of Schotten-Baumann esterification reaction.

Ⅲ Experimental Equipments and Raw Materials

Chlorization apparatus and esterification apparatus

1. Experimental equipments

The chlorization apparatus is composed of a magnetic stirrer, a three-neck round-bottom flask, a spherical condenser tube, a thermometer, a drying tube containing calcium chloride, and NaOH absorption solution.

The esterification apparatus is composed of a magnetic stirrer, an ice-water bath, a three-neck round-bottom flask, a thermometer, a spherical condenser tube, and a constant pressure funnel.

2. Raw materials

Name	Quantity	Quality	Use
Aspirin	9 g (0.05 mol)	Officinal	Reactant
Thionyl chloride	5 mL (0.069 mol)	CP	Chlorization reagent
Pyridine	1 drop	CP	Catalyst
Paracetamol	8.6 g (0.057 mol)	Officinal	Reactant
Sodium hydroxide	3.3 g (0.083 mol)	CP	Base
Anhydrous acetone	6 mL	AR	Solvent
Water	50 mL	—	Solvent

Ⅳ Operations

Operation demonstration of synthesis of acetyl salicyl chloride (video)

1. Preparation of acetyl salicyl chloride

(1) Equip the chlorization apparatus.

(2) Place 9 g of aspirin in a 100 mL three-neck round-bottom flask. Add 5 mL of $SOCl_2$ and one drop of pyridine in the flask. Swirl the flask, and heat the mixture slowly to 75 ℃ and maintain the temperature at 70~75 ℃ for 2 hours. The inverted funnel in the beaker serves as a trap to absorb the SO_2 and the HCl gases that are evolved during the reaction process.

(3) Cool the reaction mixture and transfer it to a single-neck flask. Cover the rubber stopper.

Experimental procedure of preparation of acetyl salicyl chloride

2. Preparation of benorilate

(1) Equip the esterification apparatus.

(2) Add 8.6 g of paracetamol and 50 mL of water to a 250 mL three-neck round-bottom flask. Cool the reaction mixture in an ice-water bath to 10~15 ℃. Add sodium hydroxide solution (3.3 g NaOH in 18 mL of H_2O) with a dropper

and keep the temperature at $10\sim15$ ℃. Cool the reaction mixture to $8\sim12$ ℃.

(3) Add 3 mL of anhydrous acetone to the above acyl chloride mixture and transfer the solution to the constant pressure drop funnel. Repeat the operation once more. Under strong agitation, add the acetonic solution of acetyl salicyl chloride dropwise through the constant pressure drop funnel to the above reaction mixture.

Operation demonstration of preparation of benorilate (video)

(4) Adjust the pH value to $9\sim10$. Remove the ice-water bath and keep the reaction temperature at $20\sim25$ ℃ for 2 hours.

(5) Filter the mixture by suction and wash it with cold water until the pH becomes neutral to obtain the crude product benorilate.

(6) Dry the product under an infrared lamp. Weigh the pure product and measure the melting point.

Experimental procedure of preparation of benorilate

(7) Send the finished product to the place where the teachers designated.

V Experimental Results

1. Yield

(1) Calculate the theoretical production of benorilate

$$\text{Aspirin} \longrightarrow \text{Benorilate}$$
$$M_w = 180.16 \text{ g/mol} \longrightarrow M_w = 313.3 \text{ g/mol}$$
$$0.05 \text{ mol} \longrightarrow 0.05 \text{ mol}$$

Theoretical production $= 0.05 \text{ mol} \times 313.3 \text{ g/mol} = 15.67 \text{ g}$

(2) Calculate the percent yield of benorilate

$$\text{Yield} = \frac{\text{Practical production}}{\text{Theoretical production}} \times 100\% = \frac{(\qquad)}{15.67 \text{ g}} \times 100\% = (\qquad)\%$$

2. Appearance and melting point of product

A. Appearance: _____ ;

B. m. p. :

Theoretical value: $179\sim180$ ℃

Practical value: _____ .

3. Analysis of experimental results

_____

_____

_____

_____

_____

_____

_____ .

VI Notes

1. The reaction of chlorization (the first reaction) should take place under a dry condition (the reaction environment including all the apparatus, reagents, and air must not contain water fraction). For this, the glass apparatus will be dried, a

drying tube which contains calcium chloride should be placed on the top position of the condenser.

2. It is necessary to install the toxic gas treatment apparatus, to avoid the harmful effect of toxic gas produced during the reaction.

3. The reaction mixture must be slowly heated to prevent the formation of the by-products.

4. The amount of pyridine used as a catalyst should not be excessive, otherwise the quality of the product will be affected.

5. The temperature must be controlled strictly at $70 \sim 75$ ℃, and should not exceed 80 ℃. Too low temperature is not beneficial to the reaction while thionyl chloride will be volatile when the temperature is too high.

Ⅶ Determination of Product Content

Measure by high-performance liquid chromatography method (General Rule 0512).

Chromatographic conditions: Using octadecylsilane bonded silica gel as the filler. Using water (pH adjusted to 3.5 with phosphoric acid)-methanol (44∶56) as the mobile phase. The detection wavelength is 240 nm. The injection volume is 10 μL.

Measurement method: Precisely weigh the test sample and reference solution, inject them into the liquid chromatograph separately, and record the chromatogram. Calculate based on peak area using the external standard method. (《Chinese Pharmacopoeia》 2020 Edition)

Ⅷ Discussion Questions

1. Why does not the reaction directly use aspirin and paracetamol to prepare benorilate?

2. What are the common reagents for the preparation of carboxylic chloride from carboxylic acid?

3. Why should some pyridine be added in the preparation of acetyl salicylic chloride? What will happen if pyridine is added in excess?

(By Yajing Chen)

实验四

贝诺酯的合成

背景知识

贝诺酯（Benorilate），又名扑炎痛、苯乐来、百乐来，是一种解热镇痛药。贝诺酯是一种前药，由阿司匹林和对乙酰氨基酚缩合而成，在临床上用于治疗风湿性关节炎、感冒发热和神经痛等。贝诺酯的疗效和阿司匹林相似，却有更长的作用时间及较少的副作用。贝诺酯的化学结构如图 4-1 所示。

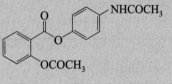

图 4-1　贝诺酯的化学结构

贝诺酯的作用机制

I　目的与要求

1. 理解制备酰氯化合物的反应原理及操作。
2. 理解拼合原理在化学结构修饰方面的应用。
3. 学习反应过程中产生的有毒气体的处理方法。
4. 掌握无水操作的方法。
5. 理解 Schotten-Baumann 酯化反应的原理。
6. 了解贝诺酯与靶标的作用方式。

II　反应原理

1. 主要反应物和产物的物理常数

名称	结构式 CAS 号	分子式 分子量	熔点或 沸点/℃	溶解度
阿司匹林	COOH OCOCH₃ 50-78-2	$C_9H_8O_4$ 180.16	m. p. 135～138	20 ℃ 水中溶解度为 3.3 g/L,20 ℃二甲基亚砜 中溶解度 100 mmol/L
邻乙酰水杨酰氯	COCl OCOCH₃ 5538-51-2	$C_9H_7O_3Cl$ 198.60	m. p. 45～49	溶于甲苯,遇水分解

实验四　贝诺酯的合成 | 31

名称	结构式 CAS 号	分子式 分子量	熔点或 沸点/℃	溶解度
二氯亚砜	$SOCl_2$ 7719-09-7	$SOCl_2$ 118.97	b. p. 79	和水反应;可溶于常用有机溶剂
吡啶	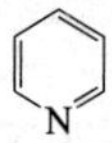 (结构式) 110-86-1	C_5H_5N 79.1	b. p. 115	可溶于水和常用有机溶剂
对乙酰氨基酚	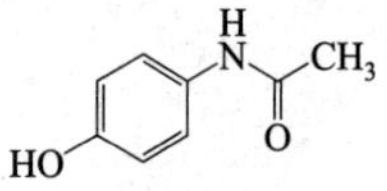 (结构式) 103-90-2	$C_8H_9NO_2$ 151.16	m. p. 168~172	20 ℃ 水中溶解度为 14 g/L,20 ℃乙醇中溶解度为 500 mmol/L,与有机溶剂混溶
贝诺酯	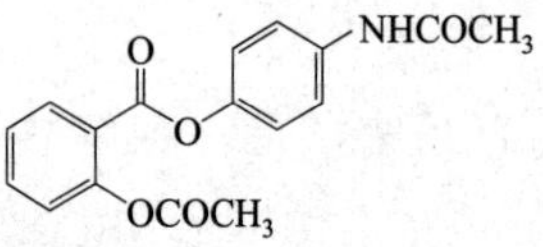 (结构式) 5003-48-5	$C_{17}H_{15}NO_5$ 313.3	m. p. 177~181	不溶于水 易溶于热的乙醇

2. 合成路线

(1) 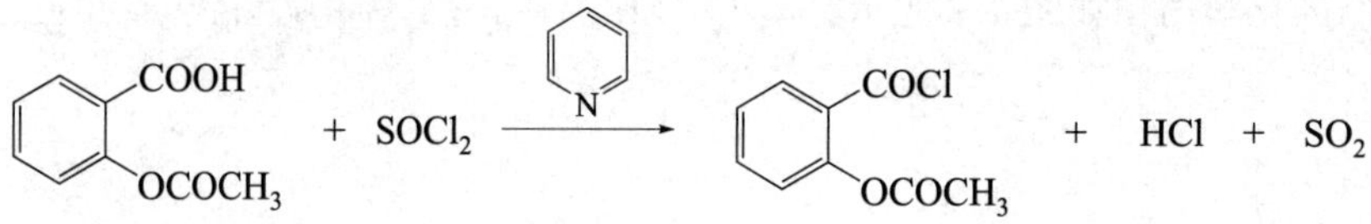 略

(2) 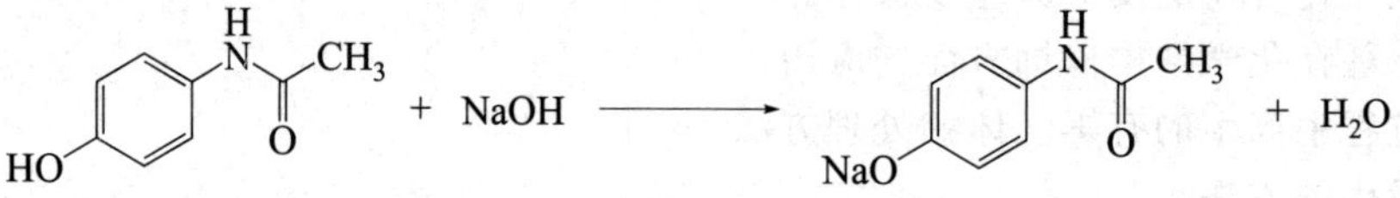 略

(3) 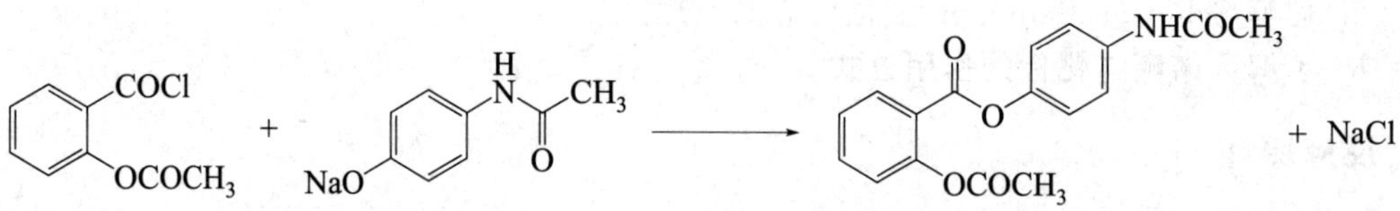 略

贝诺酯是由阿司匹林和对乙酰氨基酚缩合而成的。对乙酰氨基酚的羟基和阿司匹林的羧基发生酯化反应。在本实验中,低活性的阿司匹林首先在吡啶的催化作用下和氯化亚砜反应生成高活性的乙酰水杨酰氯;同样地,低活性的对乙酰氨基酚在碱性作用下生成高活性的钠盐,然后,高活性的乙酰水杨酰氯和对乙酰氨基酚钠盐在室温下生成贝诺酯。

安全提示:氯化亚砜和吡啶有刺激性气味,必须在通风橱中使用,它们能灼伤皮肤,刺激黏膜。氯化亚砜及酰氯遇水剧烈反应,并且产生有毒气体。

3. 知识点

氯化反应,酸性气体吸收,Schotten-Baumann 酯化反应原理。

Ⅲ 实验装置和原料

1. 实验装置

氯化实验装置由恒温磁力搅拌器、三口烧瓶、回流冷凝管、温度计、干燥管和 NaOH 吸收液组成。

酯化实验装置由恒温磁力搅拌器、冰水浴、三口烧瓶、温度计、回流冷凝管和恒压滴液漏斗组成。

氯化实验装置和酯化实验装置

2. 原料

名称	用量	规格	用途
阿司匹林	9 g (0.05 mol)	药用	反应物
氯化亚砜	5 mL (0.069 mol)	化学纯	氯化试剂
吡啶	1 滴	化学纯	催化剂
对乙酰氨基酚	8.6 g (0.057 mol)	药用	反应物
氢氧化钠	3.3 g (0.083 mol)	化学纯	碱
无水丙酮	6 mL	分析纯	溶剂
水	50 mL	—	溶剂

Ⅳ 实验操作

1. 乙酰水杨酰氯的制备

（1）搭建氯化实验装置。

（2）于干燥的 100 mL 三口烧瓶中，加入 9 g 阿司匹林、5 mL 氯化亚砜及 1 滴吡啶。缓缓加热至 75 ℃，维持 70～75 ℃，保温反应 2 h。将生成的 SO_2 和 HCl 有害气体通过长颈漏斗导入到氢氧化钠吸收液中。

（3）冷却，转移至单口烧瓶中，盖上橡胶塞。

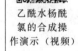

乙酰水杨酰氯的合成操作演示（视频）

2. 贝诺酯的制备

（1）搭建酯化实验装置。

（2）于干燥的 250 mL 三口烧瓶中，加入 8.6 g 对乙酰氨基酚和 50 mL 水。冰水浴中冷却混合物温度至 10～15 ℃。于 10～15 ℃缓缓加入 18 mL 氢氧化钠液（3.3 g NaOH 加水至 18 mL）。降温至 8～12 ℃。

（3）在上述制备的乙酰水杨酰氯中加入 3 mL 无水丙酮并将该丙酮溶液转移至恒压滴液漏斗中，再次向乙酰水杨酰氯储存瓶中加入 3 mL 无水丙酮并将该溶液一并转移至恒压滴液漏斗中。缓慢滴加上述制得的 6 mL 乙酰水杨酰氯无水丙酮液。

贝诺酯的制备操作演示（视频）

（4）调节 pH 至 9～10，撤去冰水浴，于 20～25 ℃搅拌反应 2 h。

（5）反应完毕，抽滤，用水洗至中性，得产品。

（6）烘干纯品，称重，计算收率，测熔点。

（7）将产物送到指导教师指定的产品回收处。

Ⅴ 实验结果

1. 收率

(1) 计算贝诺酯的理论产量

$$阿司匹林————贝诺酯$$

$$M_w = 180.16 \text{ g/mol} ————M_w = 313.3 \text{ g/mol}$$

$$0.05 \text{ mol} ————0.05 \text{ mol}$$

理论产量 $= 0.05 \text{ mol} \times 313.3 \text{ g/mol} = 15.67 \text{ g}$

(2) 计算贝诺酯的收率

$$收率 = \frac{产品实际产量}{产品理论产量} \times 100\% = \frac{(\quad\quad)}{15.67 \text{ g}} \times 100\% = (\quad\quad)\%$$

2. 产品外观与熔点

A. 外观：_____；

B. 熔点：

理论值：179～180 ℃

实测值：_____。

3. 实验结果分析

_____
_____
_____
_____
_____
_____
_____
_____。

Ⅵ 注意事项

1. 第一步氯化反应需在无水条件下操作，因此，实验前，需要将所有玻璃仪器干燥，回流冷凝管顶部需加氯化钙干燥管。

2. 因为反应会生成氯化氢和二氧化硫有毒气体，因此需要使用尾气吸收装置。

3. 为了避免副产物的生成，反应要缓慢升温。

4. 吡啶不可过量，否则影响产品的质量和产量。

5. 反应过程中，注意控制温度在70～75 ℃为佳。反应温度过低，不利于反应进行；温度太高，氯化亚砜易挥发。

Ⅶ 产物的含量测定

照高效液相色谱法（通则0512）测定。

色谱条件：用十八烷基硅烷键合硅胶为填充剂；以水（用磷酸调节 pH 值至3.5)-甲醇（44：56）为流动相；检测波长为 240 nm；进样体积 10 μL。

测定法：精密量取供试品与对照品溶液，分别注入液相色谱仪，记录色谱图。按照外标法以峰面积计算。（《中华人民共和国药典（2020年版）》）

Ⅷ 思考题

1. 为何不直接用阿司匹林和对乙酰氨基酚制备贝诺酯？

2. 由羧酸制备酰氯的常用方法有哪些？

3. 由羧酸和氯化亚砜制备酰氯时，为什么要加入少量的吡啶？吡啶的量若加多了会发生什么后果？

（陈亚静）

Experiment 5
Synthesis of Sulfacetamide Sodium

Background

The sulfanilamide derivatives of *p*-aminobenzene sulfonamide parent ring (Fig. 5-1), the earliest synthetic antibacterial drugs, play an important role in the treatment of infectious diseases with broad antibacterial spectrum, oral and rapid absorption.

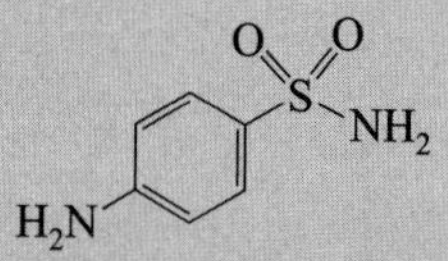

p-Aminobenzene sulfonamide 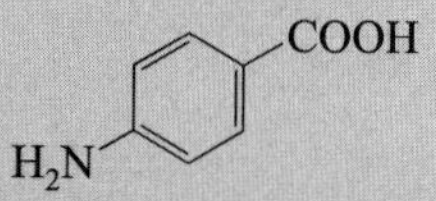   *p*-Aminobenzoic acid

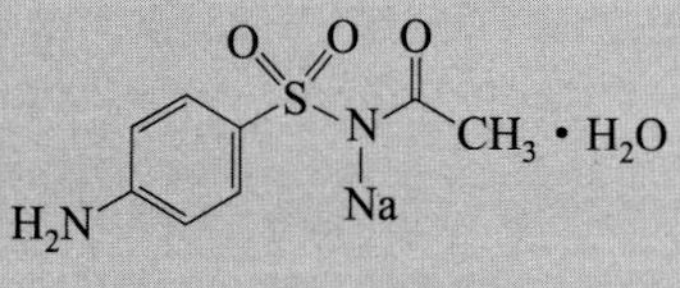

Sulfacetamide sodium

Fig. 5-1   The structure of *p*-Aminobenzene sulfonamide，*p*-Aminobenzoic acid and Sulfacetamide sodium

The mechanism of action of Sulfacetamide sodium

Ⅰ Purposes and Requirements

1. To understand the general physical and chemical properties of sulfanilamides，and to know how to purify the product using these properties.

2. To master the principle and the operation of acetylation.

3. To understand the interaction between sulfacetamide sodium and target.

Ⅱ Principle of the Reaction

1. Physical data of the main reactants and product

Name	Structure CAS No.	Formula M. Wt	b. p. or m. p. /℃	Solubility
Sulfanilamide	(structure) 63-74-1	$C_6H_8N_2O_2S$ 172.21	m. p. 165~166	Slightly soluble in cold water and ethanol; soluble in NaOH solution; Insoluble in chloroform, ether
Sulfacetamide	(structure) 144-80-9	$C_8H_{10}N_2SO_3$ 214.24	m. p. 179~184	Soluble in ethanol, slightly soluble in water or ether
Sulfacetamide Sodium	(structure) 127-56-0	$C_8H_9N_2NaO_3S \cdot H_2O$ 254.24	—	Soluble in water, slightly soluble in ethanol and acetone
Acetic anhydride	(structure) 108-24-7	$C_4H_6O_3$ 102.09	b. p. 138~139	React with water to form acetic acid and miscible with ether, chloroform and benzene

2. Synthetic route

In this reaction, the synthesis of sulfacetamide sodium is by the way that sulfacetamide is prepared by acetylation of sulfanilamide. Sulfacetamide then reacts with sodium hydroxide aqueous solution in ethanol to generate its sodium salt. There are two amino groups in the structure of sulfanilamide and diacetylated products can be produced. In this acetylation process, the issue of specificity should be considered. The pH of the reaction is very important and it is important to control the specificity of the synthesis route as well as the separation and crystallization of the final reaction product.

The dissolution of the products and by-products at different pH are shown in Table 5-1. The dissolution and precipitation of the products and by-products during the experiment are shown in Fig. 5-2. During the operation, attention should be paid to distinguishing the filtrate from the filter cake.

Table 5-1　The dissolution of the products and by-products at different pH

Name	pH=7	pH=4~5	pH<2
Sulfanilamide	Very low solubility	Sulfanilamide salt Dissolve	Sulfanilamide hydrochloride Dissolve
Sulfacetamide	Sulfacetamide sodium Dissolve	Low solubility	Sulfacetamide hydrochloride Dissolve
Diacetylation products	Diacetylation products sodium Dissolve	Low solubility	Insoluble

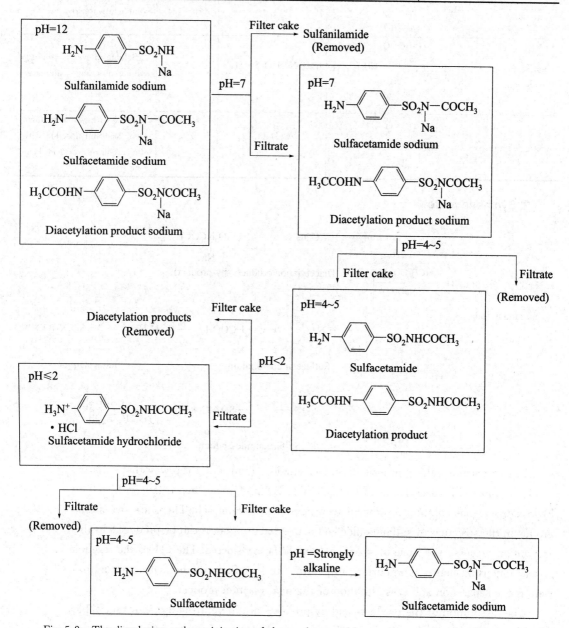

Fig. 5-2　The dissolution and precipitation of the products and by-products during the experiment

Safety Tips: Like other corrosive acids and alkalis, drops of sodium hydroxide solutions can readily cause chemical burns and may induce permanent blindness upon contact with the eyes. Thus, protective equipment, like rubber gloves, safety tips clothing and eye protection, should always be used when handling this chemical or its solution. The standard first aid method for alkali spills on the skin is, as for other corrosives, irrigation with large quantities of water for more than fifteen minutes.

3. Knowledge points

Acylation reaction, alternate dropwise addition of solution, acid-base adjustment.

Ⅲ Experimental Equipments and Raw Materials

1. Experimental equipments

The reflux apparatus is composed of a three-neck round-bottom flask, a spherical condenser tube, a magnetic stirrer, and a thermometer.

The basification apparatus is composed of a beaker, a glass rod, a dropper, and a measuring cylinder.

The reflux apparatus and the basification apparatus

2. Raw materials

Materials	Quantity	Specifications	Use
Sulfanilamide	17. 2 g (0. 1 mol)	CP	Material
Acetic anhydride	13. 6 mL (0. 14 mol)	CP	Acetylating reagent
Sodium hydroxide	22 mL (0. 11 mol)	22. 5%	Material
	12. 5 mL (0. 19 mol)	77%	Material
	Proper amount	40%	Adjusting pH
Concentrated hydrochloric acid	Proper amount	CP	Adjusting pH
Diluted hydrochloric acid	Proper amount	10%	Solvent
Active carbon (Charcoal)	0. 5 g	—	Decolorization
Sodium hydroxide-ethanol	Proper amount	5%	Generating sodium salt
Water	Proper amount	—	Dilution

Ⅳ Operations

1. The preparation of sulfacetamide

(1) Equip the reaction apparatus.

(2) Add Sulfanilamide 17. 2 g and 22. 5% sodium hydroxide aqueous solution 22 mL into a 100 mL three-necked round-bottom flask. Then stir the mixture and heat to 50 ℃.

Operation demonstration of synthesis of sulfacetamide (video)

(3) After the mixture is completely dissolved, add acetic anhydride 3. 6 mL dropwise. And then, add 2. 5 mL sodium hydroxide aqueous solution (77%) 5 minutes later and the pH of the reaction solution should be kept between 12 and 13.

(4) Add 2 mL acetic anhydride dropwise for the first time (dropper). React for 5 minutes.

(5) 2 mL 77% sodium hydroxide aqueous solution for the first time dropwise (dropper). React for 5 minutes.

(6) Then, repeat the dripping process of steps (4) and (5) for four times. During the addition of materials, the reaction temperature should be maintained at 50~55 ℃ and the pH between 12 and 13.

(7) After that, maintain the reaction mixture at 50~55 ℃ for 30 minutes with stirring.

(8) Pour the reaction mixture into a 100 mL beaker and dilute it with 20 mL water. Adjust the pH to 7 with concentrated hydrochloric acid. Then put in ice-water bath for 20~30 minutes in order to precipitate the solid.

(9) Collect the solid by suction and wash it with the proper amount of ice water. Then combine the above filtered solution and washed solution, and adjust the pH to 4~5 with concentrated hydrochloric acid. Collect the solid and dry it by suction.

(10) Dissolve the precipitate with 10% hydrochloric acid (3 times the volume of the precipitate). Add another 5 mL of water. Let the solution settle for 30 minutes and remove the undissolved solid by filtration. Next, add 0.5 g of activated charcoal to the filtrate to decolorize at room temperature. After suction filtration, adjust the pH of the filtrate (pH = 5) with 40% sodium hydroxide solution. Sulfacetamide precipitates from the solution and is collected by suction.

(11) Dry the product under an infrared lamp. Weigh the pure product and measure the melting point.

2. The preparation of sodium sulfacetamide

(1) Equip the basification apparatus.

(2) Put the above obtained sulfacetamide into a 100 mL beaker. Add 5% sodium hydroxide-ethanol solution (4 times the volume of the product), stir it at room temperature until the solid is completely dissolved and then precipitate out the solid product from the solution. Collect the solid by suction and wash it with a proper amount of ethanol.

(3) Dry the product under infrared lamp. Weigh the pure product and measure the melting point.

(4) Send the final product to the place where the teachers designated.

V Experimental Results

1. Yield

(1) Calculate the theoretical production of sulfacetamide sodium

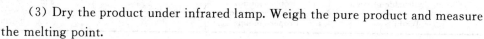

Sulfanilamide ——————— Sulfacetamide Sodium

$M_w = 172.21$ g/mol ——————$M_w = 254.24$ g/mol

0.1 mol ——————0.1 mol

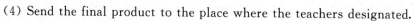

Theoretical production $= 0.1$ mol $\times 254.24$ g/mol $= 25.42$ g

(2) Calculate the percent yield of sulfacetamide sodium

$$\text{Yield} = \frac{\text{Practical production}}{\text{Theoretical production}} \times 100\% = \frac{(\quad)}{25.42 \text{ g}} \times 100\% = (\quad)\%$$

2. Appearance and melting point of product

A. Appearance: _____ ;

B. m. p. :

    Theoretical value: 179~184 ℃

    Practical value: _____ .

3. Analysis of experimental results

_____

_____

_____

_____

_____

_____

_____ .

Ⅵ Notes

1. In the experiment, different concentrations of sodium hydroxide aqueous solution are used. Careful operation is necessary.

2. Acetic anhydride and sodium hydroxide aqueous solution should be added every five minutes. After adding one of these solutions, allow it to react for 5 minutes, and then add another solution. The solution should be added drop by drop.

3. It is important to keep the pH of the solution between 12 and 13 during the reaction, otherwise the yield will be reduced.

4. Precipitate different solid products under different pH conditions. Don't mix up.

Ⅶ Determination of Product Content

Titration method: Take approximately 0.45 g of this product, weigh it accurately, and titrate it with sodium nitrite titrant (0.1 mg/L) according to the permanent stop titration method (General Rule 0701) . Every 1 mL of sodium nitrite titrant (0.1 mg/L) is equivalent to 23.62 mg of Sulfacetamide Sodium. (《Chinese Pharmacopoeia》 2020 Edition)

Ⅷ Discussion Questions

1. During the reaction, what are the solids precipitated at pH＝7 and pH＝5? What is the insoluble solid in 10% hydrochloric acid?

2. During the reaction, it is very important to adjust pH between 12 and 13, and what will happen if alkaline is too strong or too weak?

（By Lina Ding）

磺胺醋酰钠的合成

背景知识

具有对氨基苯磺酰胺结构片段（图 5-1）的磺胺类药物是应用最早的一类化学合成抗菌药，在治疗感染性疾病中起着重要作用，具有抗菌谱广、可以口服、吸收较迅速等特点。

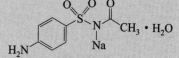

磺胺醋酰钠的作用机制

对氨基苯磺酰胺　　　　　　　对氨基苯甲酸　　　　　　　　磺胺醋酰钠

图 5-1　对氨基苯磺酰胺、对氨基苯甲酸及磺胺醋酰钠的结构

Ⅰ　目的与要求

1. 通过本实验，掌握磺胺类药物的一般理化性质，并掌握如何利用其理化性质的特点来达到分离提纯产品的目的。

2. 通过本实验操作，掌握乙酰化反应的原理。

3. 了解磺胺醋酰钠与靶标的作用方式。

Ⅱ　实验原理

1. 主要反应物、产物的物理性质

试剂名称	结构式 CAS 号	分子式 分子量	沸点或熔点 /℃	溶解性
磺胺	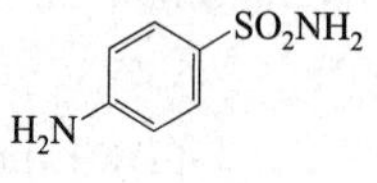 H_2N—⟨⟩—SO_2NH_2 63-74-1	$C_6H_8N_2O_2S$ 172.21	m. p. 165～166	微溶于冷水、乙醇，易溶于 NaOH 溶液，不溶于氯仿、乙醚
磺胺醋酰	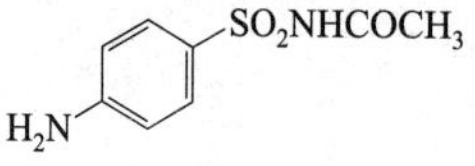 H_2N—⟨⟩—$SO_2NHCOCH_3$ 144-80-9	$C_8H_{10}N_2SO_3$ 214.24	m. p. 179～184	溶于乙醇，微溶于水或乙醚

试剂名称	结构式 CAS 号	分子式 分子量	沸点或熔点 /℃	溶解性
磺胺醋酰钠	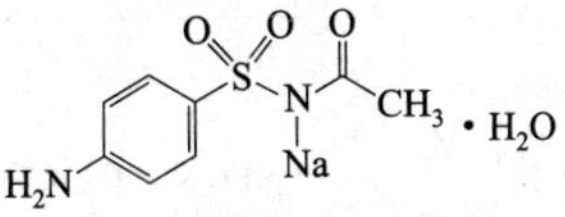 127-56-0	$C_8H_9N_2NaO_3S \cdot H_2O$ 254.24	—	易溶于水,微溶于乙醇、丙酮
乙酸酐	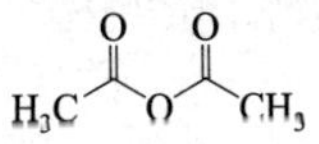 108-24-7	$C_4H_6O_3$ 102.09	b. p. 138~139	遇水反应,生成醋酸;易溶于乙醚,氯仿和苯

2. 合成路线

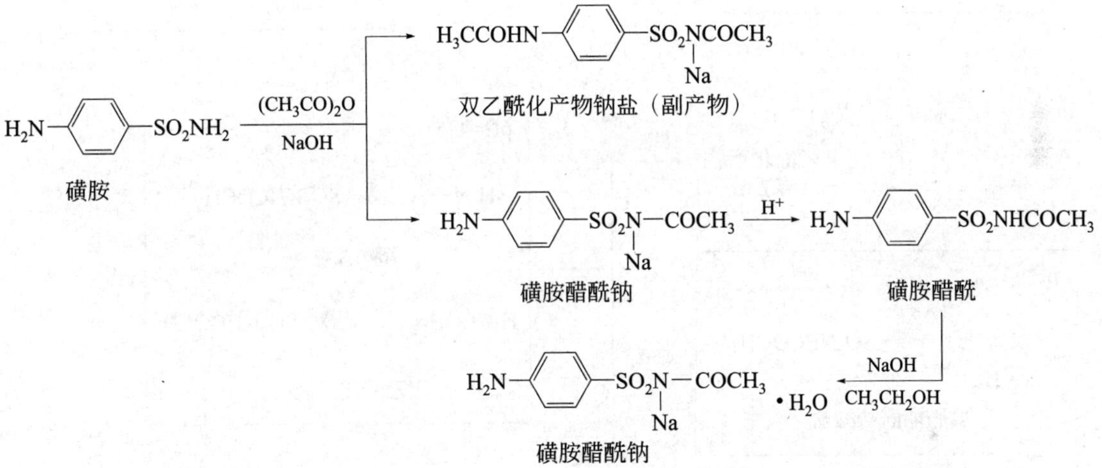

磺胺醋酰钠的合成是通过磺胺的乙酰化制备磺胺醋酰,而后在乙醇中与氢氧化钠反应制备其钠盐。在磺胺的结构中存在两个氨基,乙酰化时存在选择性问题,可生成双乙酰化产物,反应的 pH 值控制很重要,该合成路线的关键是选择性控制,以及反应终产物的分离和结晶。

反应产物及副产物在不同 pH 时的溶解情况见表 5-1。在实验过程中随溶液酸碱性溶解和析出的过程如图 5-2 所示,操作时注意将滤液和滤饼分清楚。

表 5-1 磺胺醋酰及原料、杂质的溶解度

名称	pH=7	pH=4~5	pH<2
磺胺	溶解度极小	其盐酸盐溶	其盐酸盐溶
磺胺醋酰	其钠盐溶	溶解度低	其盐酸盐溶
双乙酰化产物	其钠盐溶	溶解度低	不溶

安全提示:与其他腐蚀性酸和碱一样,氢氧化钠溶液接触皮肤后易导致化学灼伤,并且在与眼睛接触时可能引起永久失明。因此,在使用时,应始终使用防护设备,如橡胶手套、防护服和护目镜。若不慎皮肤接触,应立即用水冲洗至少 15 min。

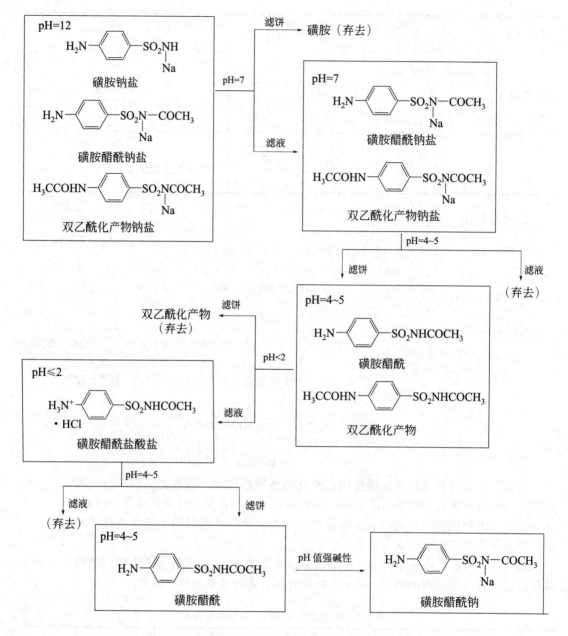

图 5-2 反应产物及副产物随溶液酸碱性溶解和析出图示

3. 知识点

酰化反应，交替滴加溶液，酸碱调节。

III 实验装置和原料

1. 实验装置

反应装置由三口烧瓶、回流冷凝管、磁力搅拌器和温度计组成。
碱化装置由烧杯、玻璃棒、滴管和量筒组成。

反应装置及
碱化装置

2. 原料

原材料名称	用量	规格	用途
磺胺	17.2 g（0.1 mol）	化学纯	原料
乙酸酐	13.6 mL（0.14 mol）	化学纯	乙酰化试剂
氢氧化钠溶液	22 mL（0.11 mol）	22.5%	原料
	12.5 mL（0.19 mol）	77%	原料
	适量	40%	调反应体系 pH 值
浓盐酸	适量	化学纯	调节体系 pH 值
稀盐酸	适量	10%	溶解沉淀
活性炭	少量	—	脱色
氢氧化钠乙醇溶液	适量	5%	成盐
水	适量	—	稀释

Ⅳ 实验操作

磺胺醋酰的
合成操作
演示（视频）

1. 磺胺醋酰的制备

（1）搭建反应装置。

（2）于 100 mL 三口烧瓶中，投入磺胺 17.2 g、22.5%氢氧化钠溶液 22 mL，开动搅拌，于水浴上加热至 50 ℃左右。

（3）待物料溶解后，滴加乙酸酐 3.6 mL，5 min 后滴加 77%的氢氧化钠溶液 2.5 mL，保持反应液 pH 在 12～13 之间。

（4）滴加 2 mL 乙酸酐，反应 5 min。

（5）滴加 2 mL 77%氢氧化钠溶液，反应 5 min。

（6）重复步骤（4）和（5）四次。加料期间，反应温度维持在 50～55 ℃，pH 值维持在 12～13。

（7）加料完毕，继续保温搅拌反应 30 min。

（8）将反应液转入 100 mL 烧杯，加水 20 mL 稀释。用浓盐酸调 pH 值至 7，于冰浴中放置 20～30 min，冷却析出固体。

（9）抽滤固体，用适量冰水洗涤。将洗液与滤液合并后用浓盐酸调 pH 值至 4～5，滤取沉淀压干。

（10）沉淀用 3 倍量的 10%的盐酸溶解，补加 5 mL 水。放置 30 min，抽滤除去不溶物，滤液加少量活性炭室温脱色后，抽滤，滤液用 40%的氢氧化钠溶液调 pH 值至 5，析出磺胺醋酰，抽滤。

（11）于红外灯下干燥，称重，测熔点。

2. 磺胺醋酰钠的制备

（1）搭建碱化装置。

（2）将以上所得的磺胺醋酰投入 100 mL 烧杯中，加入 4 倍量 5% 氢氧化钠乙醇溶液，室温搅拌至固体完全溶解，即有大量固体析出，抽滤，得到磺胺醋酰钠。

（3）烘干纯品，称重，计算收率，测熔点。

（4）将产物送到指导教师指定的产品回收处。

Ⅴ 实验结果

1. 磺胺醋酰钠收率
(1) 计算磺胺醋酰钠的理论产量

$$磺胺————磺胺醋酰钠$$
$$M_w = 172.21 \text{ g/mol} ————M_w = 254.24 \text{ g/mol}$$
$$0.1 \text{ mol} ————0.1 \text{ mol}$$
$$理论产量 = 0.1 \text{ mol} \times 254.24 \text{ g/mol} = 25.42 \text{ g}$$

(2) 计算磺胺醋酰钠的收率

$$收率 = \frac{产品实际产量}{产品理论产量} \times 100\% = \frac{(\quad\quad)}{25.42 \text{ g}} \times 100\% = (\quad\quad)\%$$

2. 产品外观与熔点
A. 外观：_____；

B. 熔点：

理论值：179～184 ℃

实测值：_____。

3. 实验结果分析

_____

_____

_____

_____

_____

_____。

Ⅵ 注意事项

1. 本实验中使用氢氧化钠溶液有多种不同浓度，实验中切勿用错。

2. 滴加乙酸酐和氢氧化钠溶液是交替进行，每滴完一种溶液后，让其反应 5 min 后，再滴入另一种溶液。滴加使用玻璃吸管加入，滴加速度以一滴一滴滴下为宜。

3. 反应中保持反应液 pH 值在 12～13 很重要，否则收率会降低。

4. 不同 pH 条件下析出固体成分不同，切勿混淆。

Ⅶ 产物的含量测定

滴定法：取本品约 0.45 g，精密称定，照永停滴定法（通则 0701），用亚硝酸钠滴定液（0.1 mol/L）滴定。每 1 mL 亚硝酸钠滴定液（0.1 mol/L）相当于 23.62mg 的磺胺醋酰钠。（《中华人民共和国药典（2020 年版）》）

Ⅷ 思考题

1. 反应过程中，pH=7 时析出的固体是什么？pH=5 时析出的固体是什么？在 10%盐酸中的不溶物是什么？

2. 反应过程中，调节 pH=12～13 是非常重要的，碱性过强或过弱会产生怎样的结果？

（丁丽娜）

Experiment 6

Synthesis of Benzocaine Intermediate Ethyl *p*-Nitrobenzoate

Background

Benzocaine is a topical anesthetic used for traumatic analgesia, ulcer pain, general itch, etc. It is not suitable for children at 2 years old or under 2 years old. It can only be used for the 2-years-old under the advice and guidance of a professional doctor after fully balancing the advantages and disadvantages under special circumstances. Benzocaine can also be used as a cosmetic ultraviolent radiation absorber. The chemical structure of benzocaine is shown in Fig. 6-1.

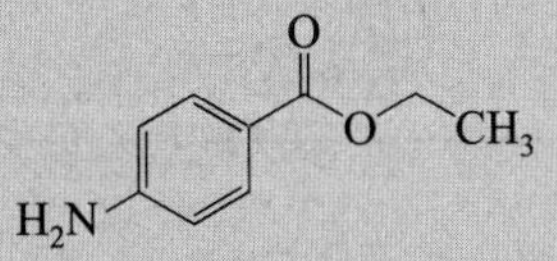

The mechanism of action of Benzocaine

Fig. 6-1   Structure of Benzocaine

The content of this experiment is the synthesis of ethyl *p*-nitrobenzoate, an intermediate of benzocaine. The obtained intermediate can be reduced to obtain the target compound benzocaine. Experiment 7 is the synthesis of Pd/TB-COF supported nanocatalysts for reduction reactions. Experiment 8 uses the product from Experiment 6 as the raw material and the product from Experiment 7 as the catalyst for the synthesis of benzocaine.

I Purposes and Requirements

1. To master the experimental principles and operations of oxidation reaction.

2. To master the experimental principles and operations of esterification reaction.

3. To understand the interaction between benzocaine and target.

II Principle of the Reaction

1. Physical data of the main reactants and product

Name	Structure CAS No.	Formula M. Wt	b. p. or m. p. / ℃	Solubility
p-Nitrotoluene	99-99-0	$C_7H_7NO_2$ 137. 13	m. p. 51. 7	Do not dissolve in water; soluble in ethanol, ether, chloroform and benzene
p-Nitrobenzoic acid	62-23-7	$C_7H_5NO_4$ 167. 13	m. p. 237~240	Slightly soluble in water; soluble in organic solvents such as ethanol
Ethyl p-nitrobenzoate	99-77-4	$C_9H_9NO_4$ 195. 17	m. p. 56~59	Soluble in ethanol and ether; insoluble in water
Benzocaine	94-09-7	$C_9H_{11}NO_2$ 165. 19	m. p. 88~90	Soluble in ethanol, ether and chloroform
Sodium dichromate dihydrate	$Na_2Cr_2O_7 \cdot 2H_2O$ 7789-12-0	$Na_2Cr_2O_7 \cdot 2H_2O$ 297. 85	m. p. 357 (anhydrous)	Soluble in water, aqueous solution is acidic; insoluble in ethanol
Concentrated sulfuric acid	H_2SO_4 7664-93-9	H_2SO_4 97. 96	—	More than the mass fraction of 70% pure H_2SO_4 aqueous solution

2. Synthetic route

p-Nitrotoluene   p-Nitrobenzoic acid

Ethyl p-nitrobenzoate   Benzocaine

The synthesis of benzocaine is started with p-nitrotoluene as a raw material. The first step is the oxidation of p-nitrotoluene by sodium dichromate to produce p-nitrobenzoic acid. The second step is an esterification reaction catalyzed by sulfuric acid to prepare ethyl p-nitrobenzoate. The target product benzocaine is finally obtained by reducing p-nitrobenzoate. The final step of the reduction reaction is virtual simulation experiment (Experiment 7 and Experiment 8).

Safety Tips: Concentrated sulfuric acid, glacial acetic acid, sodium hydroxide, and other strong acid and alkali reagents will be touched in this experiment. It should be noted that all the operations must be in ventilation. Strict compliance of operating procedures must be obeyed. You should also wear protective rubber gloves. When diluting or preparing an acid solution, acid is added to the water to avoid boiling and splashing. If sulfuric acid drops on your hand accidentally, you should immediately rinse your hand with plenty of water, and coat your hand with about 3% sodium bicarbonate solution. After the first aid treatment, you should go quickly to the nearby hospital for burn treatment to avoid further damage to the skin. If your skin contact with sodium hydroxide, you should rinse it with water for at least 15 minutes (dilute solution) or wipe your skin with a dry cloth (concentrate), then rinse it with 5%～10% magnesium sulfate, or 3% boric acid solution and then get medical treatment. If your skin contact with glacial acetic acid, you should first rinse it with water, and then thoroughly wash your skin with soap. If glacial acetic acid splashes into your eye, you should first rinse your eye with water, then wipe it with a dry cloth. If the situation is serious, you need to go to the hospital for medical treatment.

3. Knowledge points

Oxidation reaction, esterification reaction, and precautions for using concentrated sulfuric acid.

Ⅲ Experimental Equipments and Raw Materials

1. Experimental equipments

The oxidation reaction apparatus is composed of a magnetic stirrer, a three-neck round-bottom flask, a spherical condenser tube, a thermometer, and a constant pressure dropping funnel.

The esterification apparatus is composed of a magnetic stirrer, a three-neck round-bottom flask, a spherical condenser tube, a thermometer, and a drying tube.

The oxidation reaction apparatus and the esterification apparatus

2. Raw materials

Synthetic product	Raw materials			
	Name	Quantity	Quality	Use
p-Nitrobenzoic acid	$Na_2Cr_2O_7 \cdot 2H_2O$	23.6 g (0.08 mol)	CP	Oxidant
	Distilled water	130 mL	—	Solvent
	p-Nitrotoluene	8 g (0.06 mol)	CP	Reactant
	Concentrated sulfuric acid	32 mL	CP	Catalyst
	5% NaOH solution	90 mL	—	Adjusting pH
	Activated carbon	0.5 g	—	Discolouring agent
	5% Sulfuric acid	70 mL	—	Reductant

Synthetic product	Raw materials			
	Name	Quantity	Quality	Use
Ethyl p-nitrobenzoate	p-Nitrobenzoic acid	6 g (0. 036 mol)	Product prepared	Reactant
	Concentrated sulfuric acid	2 mL	CP	Catalyst
	Distilled water	100 mL	—	Solvent
	5% Na$_2$CO$_3$ solution	10 mL	—	Adjusting pH
	Absolute ethanol	24 mL	AR	Solvent

Ⅳ Operations

1. Preparation of p-nitrobenzoic acid

(1) Equip the oxidation reaction apparatus.

(2) Add 23. 6 g sodium dichromate (Na$_2$Cr$_2$O$_7$ · 2H$_2$O) and 50 mL water into a 250 mL three-necked round-bottom flask. Then, stir the solution until sodium dichromate is dissolved completely.

(3) Add 8 g p-nitrotoluene and then 32 mL concentrated sulfuric acid dropwise to the flask through the dropping funnel. After the concentrated sulfuric acid is added, start heating to maintain the reaction faint boiling for 60 minutes. There may be some white crystals of nitrotoluene precipitation in the condenser. Hence, you should turn down the condensed water to make it melt and drip.

(4) After the solution is cooled, pour the mixture into a 250 mL breaker containing 80 mL of cold water. After vacuum filtration, wash the filter cake with water until the filtrate is colorless.

(5) Dissolve the resulting filter cake with 90 mL of 5% sodium hydroxide warm solution. Filter the mixture by suction at 50 °C. Add 0. 5 g of activated carbon to the filtrate and stir the mixture for 5 ~ 10 minutes. Remove the activated carbon by hot vacuum filtration.

(6) After cooling, slowly pour the filtrate into 70 mL 5% sulfuric acid with full stirring. Following vacuum filtration, wash the solid with water. Dry the product under infrared lamp and weigh it up.

2. Preparation of ethyl p-nitrobenzoate (esterification)

(1) Equip the esterification apparatus.

(2) Add 6 g p-Nitrobenzoic acid and 24 mL of anhydride ethanol into a dry 100 mL three-necked round-bottom flask. Next, slowly add 2 mL of concentrated sulfuric acid and shake the flask to mix evenly. Heat the solution to reflux for 80 minutes.

(3) When the solution is slightly cold, pour the reaction solution into a breaker containing 100 mL of water with stirring. Collect the solid by vacuum filtration.

(4) Transfer the residue to a mortar. Grind it finely and add 10 mL 5% sodium carbonate solution. Grind it for another 5 minutes, and check the pH value (should be > 7) . After vacuum filtration, wash the solid mass with water. Dry the product under an infra-

Operation demonstration of synthesis of p-nitrobenzoic acid (video)

Experimental procedure of preparation of p-nitrobenzoic acid

Operation demonstration of synthesis of ethyl p-nitrobenzoate (video)

Experimental procedure of preparation of ethyl p-nitrobenzoate

red lamp and weigh it up.

(5) Send the finished product to the place where the teachers designated.

V Experimental Results

1. Yield

(1) Calculate the theoretical production of benzocaine in termediate

$$p\text{-Nitrotoluene} \longrightarrow \text{Ethyl } p\text{-nitrobenzoate}$$
$$M_w = 137.13 \text{ g/mol} \longrightarrow M_w = 195.17 \text{ g/mol}$$
$$0.06 \text{ mol} \longrightarrow 0.06 \text{ mol}$$

Theoretical production $= 0.06 \text{ mol} \times 195.17 \text{ g/mol} = 11.71 \text{ g}$

(2) Calculate the percent yield of benzocaine intermediate

$$\text{Yield} = \frac{\text{Practical production}}{\text{Theoretical production}} \times 100\% = \frac{(\qquad)}{11.71 \text{ g}} \times 100\% = (\qquad)\%$$

2. Appearance and melting point of product

A. Appearance: _____ ;

B. m. p. :

Theoretical value: 88~90 ℃

Practical value: _____ .

3. Analysis of experimental results

_____

_____

_____

_____

_____

_____

_____ .

Ⅵ Notes

1. In the oxidation reaction, when the residue was treated with 5% sodium hydroxide, the temperature should be maintained at about 50 ℃. When the temperature is low, sodium p-nitrobenzoate will precipitate and be filtered off.

2. Esterification reaction must be carried out under anhydrous conditions. If water goes into the reaction system, the yield will be reduced. Requirements of anhydrous operation include: 1) dry raw materials, 2) dry instrument and measuring cup, and 3) avoiding water going into the reaction flask during the reaction.

3. Ethyl p-nitrobenzoate and a small amount of unreacted p-nitrobenzoic acid are dissolved in ethanol, but not soluble in water. When the reaction is completed, the solution is poured into water. When the concentration of ethanol is diluted, ethyl p-nitrobenzoate and p-nitrobenzoic acid will precipitate. This method of separation for this product is called the dilution method.

4. The whole reaction takes place in a sequence whereby the product of the one

step will be used in the next step. So, the amount of reagent used should be calculated proportionally.

VII Discussion Questions

1. When the oxidation reaction is completed, on which chemical properties dose the separation of *p*-nitrobenzoic acid from the mixture depends?

2. Why is water-free operation needed in the esterification reaction?

(By En Zhang)

实验六

苯佐卡因中间体对硝基苯甲酸乙酯的合成

背景知识

　　苯佐卡因（Benzocaine）为局部麻醉药，用于手术后创伤止痛、溃疡痛、一般性痒等，不适用于 2 岁及 2 岁以下儿童患者，特殊情况下经充分权衡利弊后在专业医师建议和指导下才可使用。此外，苯佐卡因也可用作化妆品紫外线吸收剂。苯佐卡因的化学结构如图 6-1 所示。

苯佐卡因的作用机制

　　本实验的内容是苯佐卡因中间体对硝基苯甲酸乙酯的合成，所获得的该中间体经还原反应即可得到目标化合物苯佐卡因。实验七为还原反应所使用的 Pd/TB-COF 负载型纳米催化剂的合成，实验八以实验六的产物为原料，以实验七的产物为催化剂，进行苯佐卡因的合成。

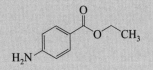

图 6-1　苯佐卡因的化学结构

Ⅰ　目的与要求

1. 掌握氧化反应的实验原理和操作。
2. 掌握酯化反应的实验原理及操作。
3. 了解苯佐卡因与靶标的作用方式。

Ⅱ　实验原理

1. 主要反应物及产物的物理常数

名称	结构式 CAS 号	分子式 分了量	沸点或熔点 /℃	溶解度
对硝基甲苯	O_2N——CH_3 99-99-0	$C_7H_7NO_2$ 137.13	m. p. 51.7	不溶于水，易溶于乙醇、乙醚、氯仿和苯
对硝基苯甲酸	O_2N——COOH 62-23-7	$C_7H_5NO_4$ 167.13	m. p. 237～240	微溶于水，能溶于乙醇等有机溶剂

名称	结构式 CAS 号	分子式 分子量	沸点或熔点 /℃	溶解度
对硝基苯 甲酸乙酯	 99-77-4	$C_9H_9NO_4$ 195.17	m. p. 56~59	易溶于乙醇和乙醚, 不溶于水
苯佐卡因	 94-09-7	$C_9H_{11}NO_2$ 165.19	m. p. 88~90	易溶于醇、醚、氯仿
重铬酸钠	$Na_2Cr_2O_7 \cdot 2H_2O$ 7789-12-0	$Na_2Cr_2O_7 \cdot 2H_2O$ 298.75	m. p. 357 (无水)	易溶于水,不溶于乙 醇,水溶液呈酸性
浓硫酸	H_2SO_4 7664-93-9	H_2SO_4 97.96	—	指质量分数大于等于 70% 的纯 H_2SO_4 的水 溶液

2. 合成路线

以对硝基甲苯为原料,首先通过重铬酸氧化制备对硝基苯甲酸,然后硫酸催化下在乙醇中反应制备对硝基苯甲酸乙酯,最后经还原得到苯佐卡因。最后一步还原反应为虚拟仿真实验(实验七和实验八)。

安全提示:本实验中会接触到浓硫酸、冰醋酸、氢氧化钠等强酸强碱试剂,在操作中注意通风,严格遵守操作规程,戴橡胶耐酸碱手套。稀释或制备酸溶液时,应把酸加入水中,避免沸腾和飞溅。如果不小心将硫酸滴在手上,立即用大量清水冲洗,并涂上浓度为 3% 左右的碳酸氢钠溶液,做完急救处理后,迅速到附近医院做灼伤处理,避免对皮肤进一步伤害。如果皮肤接触到氢氧化钠,先用水冲洗至少 15 min(稀液)/用布擦干(浓液),再用 5%~10% 硫酸镁或 3% 硼酸溶液清洗并就医;皮肤接触到冰醋酸先用水冲洗,再用肥皂彻底洗涤。若冰醋酸飞溅入眼睛,先用水冲洗,再用干布拭擦,情况严重的须送医院诊治。

3. 知识点

氧化反应,酯化反应,浓硫酸使用注意事项。

III 实验装置和原料

1. 实验装置

氧化反应装置由三口烧瓶、回流冷凝管、加热磁力搅拌器、温度计和恒压滴液漏斗组成。

酯化反应装置由磁力搅拌器、三口烧瓶、回流冷凝管、温度计和干燥管组成。

氧化反应
装置和酯化
反应装置

2. 原料

合成产物	原料			
	名称	用量	试剂级别	用途
对硝基苯甲酸	重铬酸钠（$Na_2Cr_2O_7 \cdot 2H_2O$）	23.6 g（0.08 mol）	化学纯	氧化剂
	蒸馏水	130 mL	—	溶剂
	对硝基甲苯	8 g（0.06 mol）	化学纯	原料
	浓硫酸	32 mL	化学纯	催化剂
	5% 氢氧化钠溶液	90 mL	—	调 pH 值
	活性炭	0.5 g	—	脱色
	5% 硫酸	70 mL	—	调 pH 值
对硝基苯甲酸乙酯	对硝基苯甲酸	6 g（0.036 mol）	自制	反应物
	浓硫酸	2 mL	化学纯	催化剂
	蒸馏水	100 mL	—	溶剂
	5% 碳酸钠溶液	10 mL	—	调 pH 值
	无水乙醇	24 mL	分析纯	溶剂

IV 实验操作

1. 对硝基苯甲酸的制备

（1）搭建氧化反应装置。

（2）于 250 mL 三口烧瓶中，加入 23.6 g 重铬酸钠（含两个结晶水），50 mL 水，开动搅拌。

对硝基苯甲
酸的合成
操作演示
（视频）

（3）待重铬酸钠溶解后加入 8 g 对硝基甲苯，搅拌均匀后用滴液漏斗滴加 32 mL 浓硫酸，酸加完后开动加热，保持反应微沸 60 min（反应中，冷凝管中可能有白色针状的对硝基甲苯析出，可适当关小冷凝水，使它熔融滴下）。

（4）冷却后，将反应液倾入到盛有 80 mL 冷水的 250 mL 烧杯中，抽滤，滤渣用水洗至滤液无色。

（5）所得滤渣溶于温热的 90 mL 5% 氢氧化钠溶液中，在 50 ℃ 左右抽滤，滤液加入 0.5 g 活性炭脱色（5~10 min），趁热抽滤。

（6）冷却后，在充分搅拌下，将滤液慢慢倒入 70 mL 5% 硫酸中，抽滤，洗涤，干燥得本品，计算收率。

2. 对硝基苯甲酸乙酯的制备

（1）搭建酯化反应装置。

对硝基苯甲
酸乙酯的合
成操作演示
（视频）

（2）在干燥的 100 mL 三口烧瓶中加入 6 g 对硝基苯甲酸和 24 mL 无水乙醇，分三次加入 2 mL 浓硫酸，振摇使混合均匀，装上附有氯化钙干燥管的回流冷凝管，在油浴上加热回流 80 min。

（3）稍冷，在搅拌下，将反应液倾入 100 mL 水中，抽滤。

（4）滤渣移至乳钵中，研细后，加入 10 mL 5‰碳酸钠溶液，研磨 5 min，测 pH 值（检查反应物是否呈碱性），抽滤，用水洗涤，红外灯干燥得本品，计算收率。

（5）将产物送到指导教师指定的产品回收处。

V 实验结果

1. 收率

（1）计算苯佐卡因中间体对硝基苯甲酸乙酯的理论产量

$$对硝基甲苯————对硝基苯甲酸乙酯$$

$$M_w = 137.13 \text{ g/mol} ———— M_w = 195.17 \text{ g/mol}$$

$$0.06 \text{ mol} ————0.06 \text{ mol}$$

$$理论产量 = 0.06 \text{ mol} \times 195.17 \text{ g/mol} = 11.71 \text{ g}$$

（2）计算苯佐卡因中间体对硝基苯甲酸乙酯的收率

$$收率 = \frac{产品实际产量}{产品理论产量} \times 100\% = \frac{(\quad)}{11.71 \text{ g}} \times 100\% = (\quad)\%$$

2. 产品外观与熔点

A. 外观：_____；

B. 熔点：

　　理论值：88～90 ℃

　　实测值：_____。

3. 实验结果分析

_____

_____

_____

_____

_____

_____

_____。

VI 注意事项

1. 氧化反应中，在用 5‰ 氢氧化钠处理滤渣时，温度应保持在 50 ℃ 左右，温度低，对硝基苯甲酸钠也会析出而被滤出。

2. 无水操作的要求点是：1）原料干燥无水；2）所用仪器、量具干燥无水；3）反应期间避免水进入反应瓶。

3. 对硝基苯甲酸乙酯及少量未反应的对硝基苯甲酸均溶于乙醇，但均不溶于水。反应完毕，将反应物倾入水中，乙醇的浓度变稀，对硝基苯甲酸乙酯及对硝基苯甲酸便析出，这种分离产物的方法称为稀释法。

4. 整个反应是接着上一步反应进行的，所用试剂的量需要按照比例计算后使用。

Ⅶ 思考题

1. 氧化反应完毕，依据哪些性质将对硝基苯甲酸从混合物中分离出来？
2. 酯化反应为什么需无水操作？

（张恩）

Experiment 7

Synthesis of Pd/TB–COF supported Nanocatalysts
(Virtual Simulation Experiment)

Background

Metal nanocatalyst particles generally have high activity and atomic utilization efficiency, but they are ultrafine powders with high surface energy and are in an unstable state. They are prone to aggregation during catalytic reactions (Fig. 7-1), forming secondary particles that increase the particle size and lose the characteristics of nanoparticles. Therefore, the preparation and preservation of metal nanocatalysts are a challenge.

Supported metal nanocatalysts (SMNC) are metal nanocatalysts obtained by loading noble metal nanoparticles (NP) onto a carrier through various chemical bonds such as coordination bonds. This is a very important and common type of catalyst system.

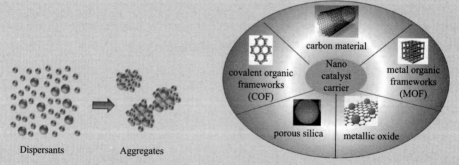

Dispersants   Aggregates

Fig. 7-1   Agglomeration of nanoparticles   Fig. 7-2   Nano catalyst carrier

Loading noble metal nanoparticles onto a carrier can effectively reduce the high surface energy of nanoparticles and enhance stability. There are various types of substances that can be used as carriers for noble metal nanoparticles, including porous silica, metal oxides, carbon materials, metal organic frameworks (MOF), covalent organic frameworks (COF), and other chemical substances (Fig. 7-2). Among them, covalent organic frameworks (COF) are a new type of crystalline porous polymer with a high specific surface area. In recent years, COF have been widely used in catalysis, gas adsorption/separation, energy storage, water splitting, and sensing. As catalyst carriers, COF have the characteristics of a crystalline state, high thermal stability, high specific surface area, wide and adjustable pore size range, diverse structural units, and low density.

Ⅰ Purposes and Requirements

1. To understand the experimental principles of ultrasonication, Soxhlet extraction, and supercritical CO_2 activation.

2. To master the preparation principle and synthesis operation of the TB-COF catalyst carrier.

3. To master the preparation principle and experimental operation of the Pd/TB-COF catalyst.

Ⅱ Principle of the Reaction

1. Physical data of the main reactants and product

Name	Structure CAS No.	Formula M. Wt	b. p. or m. p. /℃	Solubility
1,3,5-Tris (p-formylphenyl) benzene	CHO ... OHC ... CHO 118688-53-2	$C_{27}H_{18}O_3$ 390.43	m. p. 230~234	Soluble in DMF and DMSO
4,4'-Diamino biphenyl	H_2N—◯—◯—NH_2 92-87-5	$C_{12}H_{12}N_2$ 184.24	b. p. 128	Slightly soluble in water ($<$0.1 g/100 mL at 22 ℃). Easy to dissolve in boiling ethanol, acetic acid, and dilute hydrochloric acid
TB-COF	—	—	—	—
Pd/TB-COF	—	—	—	—
Trifluoromethanesulfonic acid scandium[Sc(OTf)$_3$]	$\left[F_3C-\overset{O}{\underset{O}{S}}-O^- \right]_3$ Sc^{3+} 144026-79-9	$Sc(SO_3CF_3)_3$ 492.16	$>$300	Soluble in water, ethanol, and acetonitrile

Name	Structure CAS No.	Formula M. Wt	b. p. or m. p. /℃	Solubility
Sodium chloropalladate	Na_2PdCl_4 13820-53-6	Na_2PdCl_4 294. 21	—	—
Hydrogen	H_2 1333-74-0	H_2 2. 02	b. p. —252. 8	Highly flammable and in- soluble in water

2. Synthetic route of Pd/TB-COF

The synthesis of TB-COF is carried out using aromatic aldehyde 1,3,5-tris (p-formylphenyl) benzene (TFPB) and primary amine 4, 4'-diaminobiphenyl (BND) as raw materials, and Lewis acid trifluoromethanesulfonic acid scandium $[Sc(OTf)_3]$ as catalyst. The imine type compound, namely TB-COF crude product, is obtained through nucleophilic addition and elimination reactions, and then subjected to ultrasonication, Soxhlet extraction, and supercritical CO_2 activation process to obtain light yellow powder TB-COF.

The synthesis of Pd/TB-COF is carried out using sodium chloropalladate (Na_2PdCl_4) and TB-COF as raw materials. After ultrasonication, a dispersed system is obtained. Then, hydrogen gas is used as a reducing agent to reduce sodium chloropalladate to elemental palladium. The resulting elemental palladium is then loaded onto TB-COF material in the form of ultrafine palladium nanoparticles with an average size of 1.8 nm through coordination bonds, obtaining a Pd/TB-COF supported nano catalyst (Fig. 7-3). The palladium loading of the supported palladium nanocatalyst used in this experiment is as high as 5% (mass fraction).

This experiment uses ultrasonication technology for the dispersion of TB-COF and Na_2PdCl_4/TB-COF, respectively. Ultrasonic waves can generate the phenomenon of "ultrasonic cavitation", which means that when the ultrasonic energy is high enough, "ultrasonic cavitation" can produce a local high temperature and highpressure environment of about 4000 K and 100 MPa in an instant, which can cause disturbances and phase interface update at heterogeneous interfaces. Ultrasonication refers to the process of using ultrasonic energy to change the physical, chemical, and biological properties or states of a substance, or to accelerate the rate of such changes. Ultrasonication is commonly used in nanotechnology to uniformly disperse nanoparticles in liquids.

This experiment used the Soxhlet extraction technique to remove organic impurities from the TB-COF crude product. Soxhlet extraction utilizes the reflux and siphon principles of solvents to continuously extract certain components from solid mixtures. The extracted substances are enriched in the flask, and the solvent is repeatedly used to shorten the extraction time and improve the extraction efficiency.

This experiment uses supercritical CO_2 activation technology to activate TB-COF. Supercritical CO_2 activation refers to the process of bringing CO_2 into contact with the TB-COF to be activated while in a supercritical state. Then, by

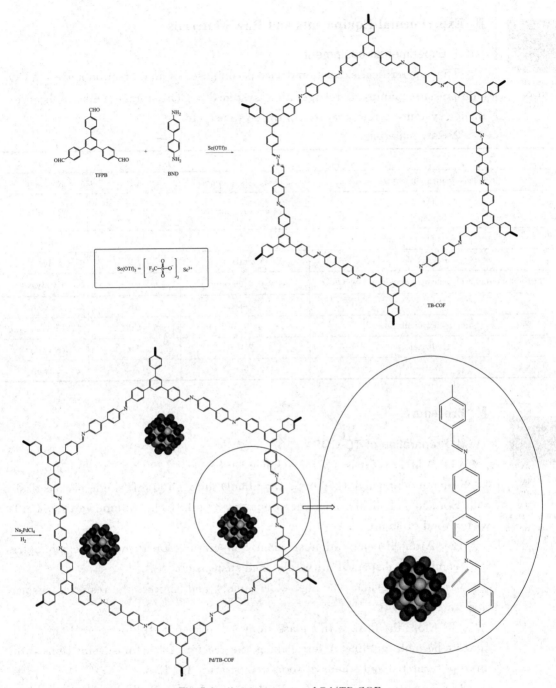

Fig. 7-3　Synthetic route of Pd/TB-COF

reducing pressure and increasing temperature, the supercritical fluid is transformed into a normal gas, completely removing impurities from the TB-COF crystal cavity and obtaining activated TB-COF.

3. Knowledge points

Nucleophilic addition-elimination reaction, reduction reaction, ultrasonication, Soxhlet extraction, and supercritical CO_2 activation.

Ⅲ Experimental Equipments and Raw Materials

Supercritical extraction device

1. Experimental equipment

The supercritical extraction device is composed of an extraction kettle, a CO_2 high-pressure pump, a refrigeration system, a CO_2 storage tank, a heat exchange system, a temperature control system, etc.

2. Raw materials

Name	Quantity	Quality	Use
1,3,5-Tris(p-formylphenyl)benzene	390 mg (0.99 mmol)	CP	Reactant
4,4′-Diamino biphenyl	276 mg (1.5 mmol)	CP	Reactant
1,2-Dichlorobenzene	24 mL	AR	Solvent
n-Butanol	6 mL	AR	Solvent
Trifluoromethanesul fonic acid scandium [Sc(OTf)$_3$]	30 mg (0.06 mmol)	CP	Catalyst
Ethanol	150 mL	AR	Solvent
Sodium chloropalladate	27.6 mg (9.39 mmol)	CP	Reactant
Hydrogen	适量	AR	Reductant
Water	2.76 mL	—	Solvent

Ⅳ Procedure

Virtual simulation experiment demonstration of preparation of TB-COF

1. Preparation of TB-COF

(1) Add 1,3,5-tris (p-formylphenyl) benzene (390 mg, 0.99 mmol) and 4, 4′-diamino biphenyl (276 mg, 1.5 mmol) into a 100 mL single-necked flask, and then add 1,2-dichlorobenzene/n-butanol 30 mL (The volume ratio is 4 : 1, with a total of 30 mL).

(2) After ultrasonication at room temperature for 10 min, the monomers were completely dispersed in the obtained suspension.

(3) Add Sc(OTf)$_3$ (30 mg, 0.06 mmol) and sonicate the resulting suspension for 1 min.

(4) Close the flask with a glass stopper and keep it still for about 10 min. The mixture becomes gel-like. After shaking the reaction flask for several times, the mixture turns red and stands at room temperature for 12 h.

(5) Transfer the mixture to a Soxhlet extractor for Soxhlet extraction, using ethanol as the solvent, at an extraction temperature of 100 ℃, and for 24 h.

Virtual simulation experiment demonstration of preparation of Pd/TB-COF

(6) Subsequently, the supercritical CO_2 activation process was carried out at a supercritical temperature of 45 ℃, a pressure of 25 MPa, and a time of 1 h to obtain 493.6 mg of TB-COF in the form of a light-yellow powder with a yield of 86%.

2. Preparation of Pd/TB-COF

(1) Add 200 mg TB-COF to 20 mL ethanol and sonicate to obtain a suspension.

(2) Add Na_2PdCl_4 aqueous solution (27.6 mg Na_2PdCl_4 dissolved in 2.76 mL water) and sonicate for 10 min.

(3) Stir the mixture at room temperature for 12 h.

(4) Filter the reaction mixture and place the filter cake and filter paper together in a supercritical extractor for supercritical CO_2 drying.

(5) The dried material is placed in a U-shaped tube and reduced in a hydrogen stream at 200 ℃ for 2 h.

(6) Stop heating, stop introducing hydrogen gas, cool down, introduce nitrogen gas to replace hydrogen gas, open the plug, remove the product, and obtain a TB-COF catalyst loaded with palladium. Quantitative completion of the reaction.

Ⅴ Experimental Results

1. Yield

The obtained Pd/TB-COF catalyst has a Pd loading of 5.0% (mass fraction), and the sample is labeled as $Pd_{5.0}$/TB-COF. The overall yield of the reaction was 86%.

2. Analysis of experimental results

_____

_____

_____

_____

_____

_____

_____.

Ⅵ Discussion Questions

1. What substances can be used as carriers for noble metal nanoparticles?

2. Regarding Pd/TB-COF catalysts, what chemical bonds are formed that allow palladium to be loaded onto TB-COF?

(By Wen Li)

Pd/TB-COF负载型纳米催化剂的合成（虚拟仿真实验）

背景知识

金属纳米催化剂具有高活性和高原子利用率，但由于其超细粉末特性和高表面能，其处于不稳定状态，容易在催化过程中发生团聚（图7-1），导致粒径增大，失去纳米颗粒特性。因此，金属纳米催化剂的制备和保存是一个重要挑战。

负载型金属纳米催化剂（supported metal nanocatalysts，SMNC）是将贵金属纳米颗粒（nanoparticles，NP）通过配位键等各种化学键负载于载体上，所获得的金属纳米催化剂，这是一类非常重要也是常见的催化剂体系。

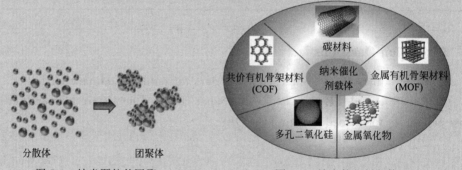

图7-1 纳米颗粒的团聚

图7-2 纳米催化剂载体

贵金属纳米颗粒负载于载体上可有效地降低纳米颗粒的高表面能，增强稳定性。可用作贵金属纳米颗粒载体的物质种类多样，包括多孔二氧化硅、金属氧化物、碳材料、金属有机骨架（metal organic framework，MOF）、共价有机骨架（covalent organic frameworks，COF）等化学物质（图7-2）。其中，共价有机骨架（COF）是一种新型的高比表面积的结晶多孔聚合物，近年来，在催化、气体吸附/分离、能量存储、水分解和传感方面得到了广泛的应用。COF作为催化剂载体具有晶态以及热稳定性高、比表面积高、孔径范围宽且可调节、结构单元多样、密度低的特性。

Ⅰ 目的与要求

1. 了解超声处理、索氏提取和超临界 CO_2 活化的实验原理。
2. 掌握 TB-COF 催化剂载体的制备原理与合成操作。
3. 掌握 Pd/TB-COF 催化剂的制备原理与实验操作。

Ⅱ 实验原理

1. 主要反应物及产物的物理常数

名称	结构式 CAS 号	分子式 分子量	沸点或 熔点/℃	溶解性
1,3,5-三(对甲酰基苯基)苯	CHO ... OHC ... CHO 118688-53-2	$C_{27}H_{18}O_3$ 390.43	m. p. 230～234	可溶于 DMF、DMSO
4,4'-二氨基联苯	H_2N ... NH_2 92-87-5	$C_{12}H_{12}N_2$ 184.24	b. p. 128	微溶于水,22 ℃水中溶解度<0.1 g/100 mL;易溶于沸乙醇、乙酸和稀盐酸
TB-COF				
Pd/TB-COF				
三氟甲烷磺酸钪 $[Sc(OTf)_3]$	$[F_3C-SO_3^-]_3$ Sc^{3+} 144026-79-9	$Sc(SO_3CF_3)_3$ 492.16	m. p. >300	溶于水、乙醇和乙腈
氯钯酸钠	Na_2PdCl_4 13820-53-6	Na_2PdCl_4 294.21	—	—
氢气	H_2 1333-74-0	H_2 2.02	b. p. —252.8	极易燃烧,难溶于水

2. Pd/TB-COF 的合成路线

TB-COF 的合成以芳香醛 1,3,5-三（对甲酰基苯基）苯（TFPB）与伯胺 4,4'-二氨基联苯（BND）为原料,以路易斯酸三氟甲烷磺酸钪 $[Sc(OTf)_3]$ 为催化剂,通过亲核加成和消去反应获得亚胺型化合物,即 TB-COF 粗品,再经超声处理、索氏提取和超临界 CO_2 活化过程获得浅黄色粉末状的 TB-COF。

Pd/TB-COF 的合成以氯钯酸钠（Na_2PdCl_4）和 TB-COF 为原料,经超声处理后获得分散体系,然后,以氢气为还原剂,将氯钯酸钠还原为单质钯,生成的单质钯随即以平均尺寸为 1.8 nm 的超细钯纳米粒形式,通过配位键负载在 TB-COF 材料上,获得 Pd/TB-COF 负载型纳米催化剂（图 7-3）。本实验所用负载型钯纳米催化剂的钯负载量高达 5%（质量分数）。

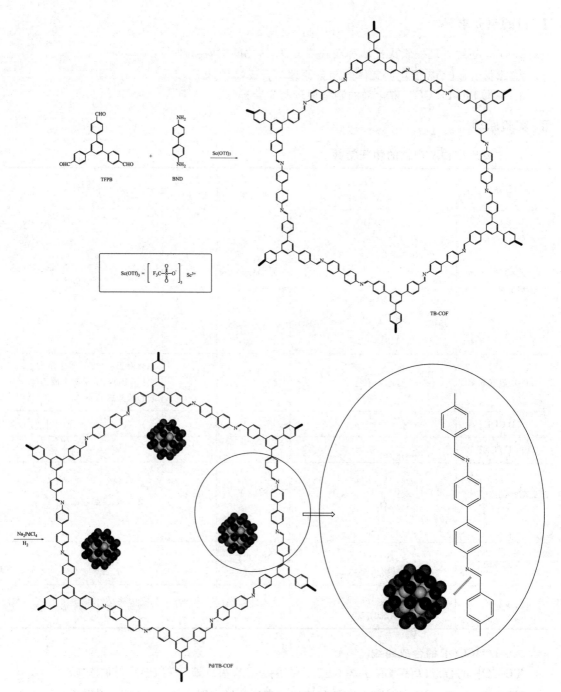

图 7-3 Pd/TB-COF 的合成路线

  本实验采用了超声处理技术，分别用于 TB-COF 和 Na_2PdCl_4/TB-COF 的分散。超声波可产生"超声空化"现象，即当超声能量足够高时，"超声空化"可产生瞬间的约 4000 K 和 100 MPa 的局部高温高压环境，可导致非均相界面间的扰动和相界面更新。超声处理是指利用超声能量使物质的一些物理、化学和生物特性或状态发生变化，或者使这种变化速度加快的处理过程。超声处理通常用于纳米技术中，以将纳米颗粒均匀地分散在液体中。

本实验也采用了索氏提取技术，用于除去 TB-COF 粗品中的有机杂质。索氏提取技术利用溶剂的回流和虹吸原理，对固体混合物中某些成分进行连续提取，将萃取出的物质富集在烧瓶中，溶剂反复利用，缩短了提取时间，并且提高了萃取效率。

本实验亦采用了超临界 CO_2 活化技术，进行 TB-COF 的活化。超临界 CO_2 活化是指在处于超临界状态时，将 CO_2 与待活化的 TB-COF 接触，然后，借助减压和升温的方法使超临界流体变成普通气体，将 TB-COF 晶体空腔中的杂质完全除去，获得活化后的 TB-COF。

3. 知识点

亲核加成-消去反应，还原反应，超声处理，索氏提取，超临界 CO_2 活化。

Ⅲ 实验装置和原料

超临界
萃取装置

1. 实验装置

超临界萃取装置由萃取釜、CO_2 高压泵、制冷系统、CO_2 贮罐、换热系统、温度控制系统等组成。

2. 原料

名称	用量	规格	用途
1,3,5-三(对甲酰基苯基)苯	390 mg(0.99 mmol)	化学纯	反应物
4,4′-二氨基联苯	276 mg(1.5 mmol)	化学纯	反应物
1,2-二氯苯	24 mL	分析纯	溶剂
正丁醇	6 mL	分析纯	溶剂
三氟甲烷磺酸钪	30 mg(0.06 mmol)	化学纯	催化剂
乙醇	150 mL	分析纯	溶剂
氯钯酸钠	27.6 mg(9.39 mmol)	化学纯	反应物
氢气	适量	分析纯	还原剂
水	2.76 mL	—	溶剂

Ⅳ 实验操作

TB-COF 制备
的虚拟仿真
实验演示

1. TB-COF 的制备

（1）将 1,3,5-三（对甲酰基苯基）苯（390 mg，0.99 mmol）和 4，4′-二氨基联苯（276 mg，1.5 mmol）装入 100 mL 单口烧瓶中，然后加入 1,2-二氯苯/正丁醇（体积比 4∶1，共 30 mL）。

（2）所得悬浮液在室温下进行超声处理 10 min 后，单体完全分散。

（3）加入 Sc(OTf)$_3$（30 mg，0.06 mmol），得到的悬浮液超声处理 1 min。

（4）用玻璃塞封闭烧瓶并保持静止约 10 min，混合物变成凝胶状，摇晃反应瓶几次后，混合物变成红色，室温静置 12 h。

（5）将混合物转移到索氏提取器中进行索氏提取，溶剂为乙醇，提取温度为 100 ℃，提取时间为 24 h。

（6）随后进行超临界 CO_2 活化，超临界的温度为 45 ℃，压力为 25 MPa，时间为 1 h，获得浅黄色粉末状的 TB-COF 493.6 mg，收率 86%。

Pd/TB-COF
制备的虚拟
仿真实验演示

2. Pd/TB-COF 的制备

(1) 将 200 mg TB-COF 加入 20 mL 乙醇中，超声处理得到悬浮液。

(2) 加入 Na_2PdCl_4 水溶液（27.6 mg Na_2PdCl_4 溶于 2.76 mL 水中），超声波处理 10 min。

(3) 在室温下搅拌混合物 12 h。

(4) 将反应混合物过滤，将滤饼和滤纸一起置于超临界萃取仪，进行超临界 CO_2 干燥。

(5) 干燥后的材料置于 U 形管中，200 ℃下在氢气流中还原 2 h。

(6) 停止加热，停止通入氢气，降温，通入氮气置换氢气，打开塞子，取出产品，获得负载钯的 TB-COF 催化剂。反应定量完成。

V 实验结果

1. 收率

所获得的 Pd/TB-COF 催化剂，Pd 负载量为 5.0%（质量分数），样品标记为 $Pd_{5.0}$/TB-COF。反应总收率为 86%。

2. 实验结果分析

_____

_____

_____

_____

_____

_____

_____ 。

VI 思考题

1. 哪些物质可用作贵金属纳米粒子载体？

2. Pd/TB-COF 催化剂中钯通过哪些化学键负载在 TB-COF 上？

（李雯）

Experiment 8

Synthesis of Benzocaine
(Virtual Simulation Experiment)

Background

In the development history of local anesthetic, the first drug obtained through chemical synthesis was benzocaine. The early synthesis of benzocaine used ethyl p-nitrobenzoate as the raw material and iron powder as the reductant, but this method is explicitly phased out by the "Guiding Catalogue for Industrial Structure Adjustment (2005 Edition)" issued by the National Development and Reform Commission. At present, the synthesis of benzocaine mostly adopts the hydrogenation reduction method and the catalytic hydrogen transfer method.

This experiment is the synthesis of benzocaine, using ethyl p-nitrobenzoate as the raw material and hydrogen or ammonium formate as the hydrogen source, respectively, to obtain the target substance through hydrogenation reduction method or catalytic hydrogen transfer method.

The hydrogenation reduction method has the advantages of easy operation, high atomic economy, clean and green. Commonly used catalysts include Raney nickel, platinum, palladium, and rhodium. To improve the catalytic performance of the catalyst, metal catalysts are often loaded on porous materials such as activated carbon, such as palladium carbon catalysts. The catalytic activity of palladium carbon catalysts is mainly related to factors such as the loading amount, particle size, and dispersion degree of palladium metal.

Hydrogen has unique properties. The explosion limit of hydrogen is 4.0% to 75.6% (volume fraction). When hydrogen is mixed with air and the volume ratio of hydrogen is within the range of 4.0% to 75.6%, it can ignite and explode due to factors such as discharge, impact, friction, open flame, hot air flow, lightning induction, electromagnetic radiation, etc. In addition, hydrogen is the smallest atom in nature with extremely strong permeability. Under high temperature and pressure conditions, hydrogen atoms can easily enter the lattice of metals and regenerate hydrogen molecules in the lattice defects of metals. As the volume of hydrogen molecules is 26 times than that of hydrogen atoms, the generated hydrogen molecules will generate a pressure of up to 100 MPa inside the metal, leading to defects and delayed cracks in the metal material, which is known as hydrogen embrittlement. Due to the explosive and hydrogen embrittlement properties of hydrogen, the hydrogenation reduction method poses high risks.

The catalytic hydrogen transfer method refers to the reaction in which hydrogen atoms are transferred from a hydrogen donor compound to a reaction substrate under the action of a catalyst. Catalytic hydrogen transfer reaction is a multiphase catalytic reduction reaction that can be used for the reduction of carbon-carbon double bonds, carbonyl groups, sulfur-containing unsaturated bonds (sulfonic acid groups, sulfonyl chloride groups), and nitrogen-containing unsaturated bonds (azide groups, azo groups, imino groups, carbon-nitrogen double bonds, nitro groups). Common catalysts include palladium carbon, palladium black, Raney nickel, etc. Common hydrogen donors include formic acid and its salts (such as ammonium formate), alcohols (such as isopropanol), hydrazine hydrate, unsaturated hydrocarbons (such as cyclohexene, tetrahydropyrrole), and triethylsilane.

The catalytic hydrogen transfer method does not require special hydrogen storage and hydrogenation reaction equipment, has mild conditions, and has the advantages of not involving hydrogen storage, not requiring pressurization equipment, and being scalable. It is an environmentally friendly reduction method, and some reactions have achieved large-scale preparation applications. The catalytic hydrogen transfer method holds a certain position in drug synthesis.

I Purposes and Requirements

1. To master the properties of hydrogen, installation and operation of hydrogenation kettle, and experimental operation of nitrogen displacement.

2. To master the experimental principles and operations of the hydrogenation reduction method.

3. To master the experimental principles and operations of the catalytic hydrogen transfer method

4. To understand the experimental procedures of thin layer chromatography (TLC).

5. To understand the analytical methods of nuclear magnetic resonance hydrogen spectrum.

Ⅱ Principle of the Reaction

1. Physical data of the main reactants and product

Name	Structure CAS No.	Formula M. Wt	b. p. or m. p. /℃	Solubility
Ethyl *p*-nitrobenzoate	99-77-4	$C_9H_9NO_4$ 195.17	m. p. 56~59	Soluble in ethanol and e-ther, insoluble in water
Benzocaine	94-09-7	$C_9H_{11}NO_2$ 165.19	m. p. 88~90	Soluble in alcohol, ether and chloroform
5%Pd/TB-COF	—	2128.40	—	—
Hydrogen	H_2 1333-74-0	H_2 2.02	b. p. —252.8	Highly flammable and in-soluble in water
10% Pd/C	10%Pd/C 7440-05-3	—	m. p. 1554	—
Ammonium formate	HCOONH$_4$ 540-69-2	CH_5NO_2 63.06	m. p. 116	Soluble in water, alcohol, and ammonia solution

2. Synthetic route

(1) Hydrogenation reduction method

In this experiment, hydrogen gas was used as the reductant, and ethyl *p*-nitrobenzoate was reduced under Pd/C or Pd/TB-COF catalysis to obtain the target compound benzocaine.

The speculated reaction mechanism is that ethyl *p*-nitrobenzoate is sequentially reduced to nitroso compounds, *N*-alkylhydroxylamine compounds, and ethyl *p*-aminobenzoate. During the reaction process, various impurities may be generated, including oxidized azo impurities, azo impurities, and hydrogenated azo impurities.

Ethyl *p*-nitrobenzoate → Nitroso compound → *N*-alkylhydroxylamine compound → Ethyl *p*-aminobenzoate

$$\text{Ethyl } p\text{-nitrobenzoate} \xrightarrow[\text{H}_2/\text{Pd/C}]{[\text{H}]} \text{Nitroso compound} \xrightarrow[\text{H}_2/\text{Pd/C}]{[\text{H}]} \text{N-alkylhydroxylamine compound} \xrightarrow[\text{H}_2/\text{Pd/C}]{[\text{H}]} \text{Ethyl } p\text{-aminobenzoate}$$

Oxidized azo impuritie

Hydrogenated azo impuritie

Azo impuritie

Safety tips： If hydrogen gas is directly filled into the reaction kettle without nitrogen replacement，an explosion may occur upon heating.

（2）Catalytic hydrogen transfer method

$$\text{Ethyl } p\text{-nitrobenzoate} + \text{HCO}_2\text{NH}_4 \xrightarrow[\text{Anhydrous ethanol}]{\text{Pd/C}} \text{Ethyl } p\text{-aminobenzoate}$$

In this experiment，ammonium formate was used as a reductant. In the presence of Pd/C，ammonium formate decomposed to generate atomic hydrogen，which reduced ethyl *p*-nitrobenzoate to the target compound benzocaine.

3. Knowledge points

Hydrogenation reduction method，catalytic hydrogen transfer method，reduction reaction mechanism，explosive and hydrogen embrittlement properties of hydrogen.

The hydrogenation reduction reaction device and the catalytic hydrogen transfer reaction device

Ⅲ Experimental Equipments and Raw Materials

1. Experimental equipment

The hydrogenation reduction reaction device is composed of a high-pressure reactor，a H_2 storage tank，a N_2 storage tank，etc.

The catalytic hydrogen transfer reaction device is composed of a three-necked round-bottom flask，a magnetic stirrer，a spherical condenser tube，etc.

2. Raw materials

Synthetic product	Raw materials			
	Name	Quantity	Quality	Use
Hydrogenation reduction method of Pd/C	Ethyl p-nitrobenzoate	1. 95 g (0. 01 mol)	Experimental product	Reactant
	10%Pd/C	0. 2 g	—	Catalyst
	Ethanol	20 mL	AR	Solvent
	H₂	appropriate amount	AR	Reductant
Hydrogenation reduction method of Pd/TB-COF	Ethyl p-nitrobenzoate	64 mg (0. 33 mmol)	Experimental product	Reactant
	5%Pd/TB-COF	1. 4 mg	CP	Catalyst
	Ethanol	3 mL	AR	Solvent
	H₂	appropriate amount	AR	Reductant
Catalytic hydrogen transfer method	Ethyl p-nitrobenzoate	1. 95 g (0. 01 mmol)	Experimental product	Reactant
	10%Pd/C	0. 1 g	—	Catalyst
	Ethanol	30 mL	AR	Solvent
	Ammonium formate	2. 27 g (36 mmol)	CP	Reductant

Ⅳ Operations

1. The properties of hydrogen and hydrogenation equipment

(1) Equip the experimental apparatus.

(2) Learn the properties of hydrogen and hydrogenation equipment according to the prompts.

Virtual simulation experiment demonstration of the properties of hydrogen

(3) Follow the prompts to replace nitrogen in the reactor. It should be noted that three nitrogen replacements are required before introducing hydrogen gas. If hydrogen gas is directly injected into the high-pressure reactor without nitrogen replacement or the high-pressure nut is not tightened, an explosion will occur and the experiment will fail.

2. Preparation of benzocaine by Pd/C hydrogenation reduction method

(1) Equip the experimental apparatus.

(2) Add 20 mL of ethanol, 1. 95 g of ethyl p-nitrobenzoate, and 0. 2 g of 10% Pd/C to the reaction kettle. Stir and dissolve, seal.

(3) Perform nitrogen replacement.

(4) Perform hydrogen replacement.

Virtual simulation experiment demonstration of Pd/C hydrogenation reduction method

(5) Adjust the hydrogen pressure to 1 atm (0. 1 MPa) and react at 45 ℃ for 5 h.

(6) Reaction complete, stop heating, cool down, close the intake switch, and open the exhaust valve to release pressure.

(7) Perform nitrogen replacement.

(8) Open the reaction kettle.

(9) The sample was analyzed by high-performance liquid chromatography (HPLC) with a yield of 89. 4%.

Virtual simulation experiment demonstration of Pd/TB-COF hydrogenation reduction method

3. Preparation of benzocaine by Pd/TB-COF hydrogenation reduction method

(1) Equip the experimental apparatus.

(2) Add 3 mL of ethanol, 0.064 g of ethyl p-nitrobenzoate, and 0.0014 g of 5% Pd/TB-COF to the reaction kettle. Stir and dissolve, seal.

(3) Perform nitrogen replacement.

(4) Perform hydrogen replacement.

(5) Adjust the hydrogen pressure to 20 atm (2 MPa) and react at 40 ℃ for 3 h. Record the pressure and temperature changes during the reaction process.

(6) Reaction complete, stop heating, cool down, close the intake switch, and open the exhaust valve to release pressure.

(7) Perform nitrogen replacement.

(8) Open the reaction kettle.

(9) The sample was analyzed by high-performance liquid chromatography (HPLC) with a yield of 99.0%.

4. Preparation of benzocaine by catalytic hydrogen transfer method

(1) Equip the experimental apparatus.

(2) Weigh 1.95 g of ethyl p-nitrobenzoate and 2.27 g of ammonium formate into a three-necked round-bottom flask, and add 30 mL of anhydrous ethanol.

Virtual simulation experiment demonstration of catalytic hydrogen transfer method

(3) Set the reaction temperature to 25 ℃. Start stirring.

(4) Weigh 0.1 g of 10% Pd/C and add it to the three-necked round-bottom flask through a feeding funnel.

(5) After stirring at 25 ℃ for 1 h, use capillary sampling to perform thin-layer chromatography (TLC) analysis (The TLC-developing agent is petroleum ether : ethyl acetate=4 : 1).

(6) After the reaction is complete, filter out the solid and wash the filter residue with 200 mL of ethanol. The filtrate is used for further post-treatment.

(7) Evaporate the filtrate using a rotary evaporator to obtain 1.54 g of white solid. The white solid is benzocaine with a yield of 93.3%.

Ⅴ Experimental Results

1. Yield

(1) The yield of benzocaine obtained by Pd/C hydrogenation reduction method is 89.4%.

(2) The yield of benzocaine obtained by Pd/TB-COF hydrogenation reduction method is 99.0%.

(3) The yield of benzocaine obtained by catalytic hydrogen transfer method is 93.3%.

2. Appearance and melting point of product

A. Appearance：_____；

B. m. p. ：

Theoretical value：88～90 ℃；

Practical value：87～89 ℃.

3. Nuclear magnetic resonance hydrogen spectrum

^{1}H NMR （300 MHz，CDCl$_3$） δ：1.3（3H，t），4.1（2H，s），4.3（2H，m），6.6（2H，d），7.8（2H，d）。

4. Analysis of experimental results

_____

_____

_____

_____

_____

_____

_____.

Ⅶ Notes

1. The color of the hydrogen gas cylinder is dark green and the font is red. The paint color and lettering should be kept vivid. Hydrogen gas cylinders should be stored in a cool and ventilated warehouse, with a temperature not exceeding 30 ℃. They should be kept away from sources of fire and heat, and protected from direct sunlight; Hydrogen gas cylinders should be stored separately from oxygen, compressed air, halogens (fluorine, chlorine, bromine), oxidants, etc. and mixed storage and transportation should be avoided; Hydrogen gas cylinders, hydrogenation kettles, and their pipelines should undergo regular safety inspections, including visual inspection, fixed-point wall thickness measurement, timed wall temperature measurement, and analysis of corrosive medium composition. Methods such as nitrogen gas sealing, non-destructive testing of the reactor inner wall, and macroscopic inspection of the inner wall should be adopted, with a focus on inspecting the weld area, weld overlay layer, bolts, nuts, washers, and internal and external support structures of the container. If necessary, measures such as airtight or hydrostatic testing should be taken to ensure the safe use of the hydrogenation reactor. The occurrence of hydrogen embrittlement in steel cylinders is related to multiple factors, and the most important measure to control hydrogen embrittlement should be to limit the steel grade, control the type and content of impurities contained, and control the tensile strength of the steel (σ_b＜882 MPa) .

2. When installing the nuts of the hydrogenation kettle, pay attention to tighening the nuts according to the diagonal principle. The main reason for doing so is to avoid uneven force and explosion. During the operation of the hydrogenation reactor, the operators should strictly follow the process operating procedures and ensure that the reaction temperature and pressure are stable. A reasonable start-up and shutdown plan should be prepared before the start-up and shutdown process, and an appropriate dehydrogenation process should be added during shutdown to avoid emergency pressure relief and cooling. When replacing hydrogen, it is strictly prohibited to directly replace air with hydrogen. If hydrogen leaks or explodes, the gas source should be immediately cut off.

3. The significance of nitrogen replacement is that nitrogen is chemically inert and not easily reacted with other substances. Using nitrogen to replace the air in the pipeline can prevent the formation of flammable mixtures of hydrogen and oxygen in the air，thereby avoiding internal combustion or explosions.

Ⅶ Discussion Questions

1. Dissolve 0.043 g of benzocaine in 0.5 mL of deuterated chloroform，and use a 300 MHz nuclear magnetic resonance instrument to measure the nuclear magnetic hydrogen spectrum as shown in the following figure (indicating the chemical shift of the peak and the hydrogen number). Analyze the ^{1}H NMR spectrum of benzocaine.

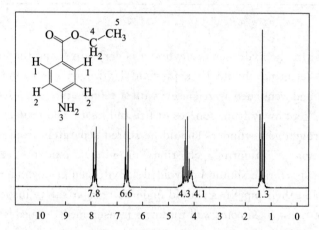

The hydrogen number corresponding to the peak with a chemical shift of 7.8 is (　　);

The hydrogen number corresponding to the peak with a chemical shift of 6.6 is (　　);

The hydrogen number corresponding to the peak with a chemical shift of 4.3 is (　　);

The hydrogen number corresponding to the peak with a chemical shift of 4.1 is (　　);

The hydrogen number corresponding to the peak with a chemical shift of 1.3 is (　　).

2. Provide examples to illustrate the application of hydrogenation reduction method in drug synthesis.

(By Wen Li)

实验八
苯佐卡因的合成（虚拟仿真实验）

背景知识

局部麻醉药发展史上，第一个实现全合成的药物为苯佐卡因。早期苯佐卡因的合成，以对硝基苯甲酸乙酯为原料，铁粉为还原剂，该法被国家发展改革委发布的《产业结构调整指导目录（2005年本）》规定为明令淘汰或立即淘汰的工艺。目前，苯佐卡因的合成多采用加氢还原法和催化氢转移法。

本实验为苯佐卡因的合成，以对硝基苯甲酸乙酯为原料，分别以氢气或者甲酸铵为氢源，通过加氢还原法或催化氢转移法获得目标物。

加氢还原法具有操作简便、原子经济性高和清洁绿色的优点，常用催化剂包括雷尼镍、铂、钯和铑，为提高催化剂催化性能，常将金属催化剂负载在活性炭等多孔物质上，如钯碳催化剂。钯碳催化剂的催化活性主要与钯金属的负载量、颗粒大小、分散程度等因素有关。

氢气具有独特的性质。氢气的爆炸极限是4.0%～75.6%（体积分数），即氢气与空气混合时，氢气体积占比在4.0%～75.6%时，遇放电、撞击、摩擦、明火、热气流、雷电感应、电磁辐射等因素，可被引燃进而发生爆炸。此外，氢是自然界半径最小的原子，渗透能力极强，在高温高压条件下，氢原子很容易进入金属的晶格中，并在金属的晶格缺陷中重新生成氢气分子，由于氢气分子的体积是氢原子的26倍，因此，生成的氢气分子会在金属内部产生高达100 MPa的压力，导致金属材料的缺陷和延迟裂纹，这种现象称为氢脆现象。由于氢气具有易爆和氢脆性质，加氢还原法存在较高的危险性，操作要求高。

催化氢转移法是指在催化剂的作用下，氢原子由氢供体化合物转移到反应底物的反应。催化氢转移反应是一种多相催化还原反应，可用于碳碳双键、羰基、含硫不饱和键（磺酸基、磺酰氯基）、含氮不饱和键（叠氮基、偶氮、亚氨基、碳氮双键、硝基）的还原。常见的催化剂包括钯碳、钯黑、雷尼镍等，常见的氢供体包括甲酸及其盐类（如甲酸铵）、醇类（如异丙醇）、水合肼、不饱和烃类（如环己烯、四氢吡咯）和三乙基硅烷等。

催化氢转移法不需要特殊的氢气贮存和氢化反应设备，条件温和，具有不涉及氢气储存、不需要加压设备和可规模化制备的优点，是一种环境友好的还原方法，部分反应已经实现规模化制备应用，在药物合成上占有一定的地位。

I 目的与要求

1. 掌握氢气的性质、氢化釜的安装操作和氮气置换实验操作。
2. 掌握加氢还原法的实验原理和实验操作。
3. 掌握催化氢转移法的实验原理和实验操作。
4. 了解薄层色谱法（TLC）的实验操作。
5. 了解核磁共振氢谱的解析方法。

II 实验原理

1. 主要反应物及产物的物理常数

名称	结构式 CAS 号	分子式 分子量	沸点或 熔点/℃	溶解性
对硝基苯甲酸乙酯	 99-77-4	$C_9H_9NO_4$ 195.17	m. p. 56～59	易溶于乙醇和乙醚,不溶于水
苯佐卡因	 94-09-7	$C_9H_{11}NO_2$ 165.19	m. p. 88～90	易溶于醇、醚、氯仿
5%Pd/TB-COF	—	2128.40	—	—
氢气	H_2 1333-74-0	H_2 2.02	b. p. —252.8	极易燃烧,难溶于水
10%钯碳	10%Pd/C 7440-05-3	—	m. p. 1554	—
甲酸铵	$HCOONH_4$ 540-69-2	CH_5NO_2 63.06	m. p. 116	溶于水、醇、氨水

2. 合成路线

（1）加氢还原法

本实验以氢气为还原剂，对硝基苯甲酸乙酯分别在 Pd/C 或 Pd/TB-COF 催化下发生还原反应，得到目标物苯佐卡因。

推测的反应机理为：对硝基苯甲酸乙酯依次还原为亚硝基化合物、N-烃基羟胺化合物和对氨基苯甲酸乙酯，反应过程中，可能生成多种化合物，包括氧化偶氮化合物、偶氮化合物和氢化偶氮化合物。

反应路线图

对硝基苯甲酸乙酯 $\xrightarrow[H_2/Pd/C]{[H]}$ 亚硝基苯甲酸乙酯 $\xrightarrow[H_2/Pd/C]{[H]}$ N-烃基羟胺化合物 $\xrightarrow[H_2/Pd/C]{[H]}$ 对氨基苯甲酸乙酯（苯佐卡因）

氧化偶氮化合物（杂质）

氢化偶氮化合物（杂质）

偶氮化合物（杂质）

安全提示：未经氮气置换，直接向反应釜内通入氢气，加热后会发生爆炸。

（2）催化氢转移法

$$\text{对硝基苯甲酸乙酯} + HCO_2NH_4 \xrightarrow[\text{无水乙醇}]{Pd/C} \text{对氨基苯甲酸乙酯}$$

本实验以甲酸铵为还原剂，甲酸铵在 Pd/C 存在下，分解生成氢原子，将对硝基苯甲酸乙酯还原为目标物苯佐卡因。

3. 知识点

加氢还原法，催化氢转移法，还原反应机理，氢气易爆性和氢脆性质。

Ⅲ 实验装置和原料

1. 实验装置

加氢还原法反应装置由高压釜、H_2 贮罐、N_2 贮罐等组成。

催化氢转移法反应装置由三口烧瓶、磁力搅拌器、回流冷凝管等组成。

2. 原料

加氢还原法和催化氢转移法反应装置

合成方法	原料			
	名称	用量	试剂级别	用途
Pd/C 催化加氢还原法	对硝基苯甲酸乙酯	1.95 g(0.01 mol)	自制	反应物
	10%Pd/C	0.2 g	—	催化剂
	乙醇	20 mL	分析纯	溶剂
	H_2	适量	分析纯	还原剂
Pd/TB-COF 催化加氢还原法	对硝基苯甲酸乙酯	64 mg(0.33 mmol)	自制	反应物
	5% Pd/TB-COF	1.4 mg	化学纯	催化剂
	乙醇	3 mL	分析纯	溶剂
	H_2	适量	分析纯	还原剂

合成方法	原料			
	名称	用量	试剂级别	用途
催化氢转移法	对硝基苯甲酸乙酯	1.95 g(0.01 mmol)	自制	反应物
	10%Pd/C	0.1 g	—	催化剂
	乙醇	30 mL	分析纯	溶剂
	甲酸铵	2.27 g(36 mmol)	化学纯	还原剂

氢气性质
虚拟仿真
实验演示

Ⅳ 实验操作

1. 氢气的性质与氢化装置

（1）搭建实验装置。

（2）按照提示学习氢气的性质和氢化装置。

（3）按照提示进行反应器的氮气置换。注意通入氢气前，需进行三次氮气置换，未经氮气置换或者高压螺母未拧紧，直接向高压釜通入氢气，将出现爆燃现象，实验失败。

Pd/C 催化
加氢还原法
虚拟仿真
实验演示

2. Pd/C 催化加氢还原法制备苯佐卡因

（1）搭建实验装置。

（2）在反应釜中加入 20 mL 乙醇，1.95 g 对硝基苯甲酸乙酯和 0.2 g 10% Pd/C。搅拌溶解，密封。

（3）进行氮气置换。

（4）进行氢气置换。

（5）调节氢气压力为 1 atm（0.1 MPa），45 ℃下反应 5 h。

（6）反应完毕，停止加热、冷却、关闭进气开关、打开排气阀泄压。

（7）进行氮气置换。

（8）打开反应釜。

（9）取样，经高效液相色谱法（HPLC）检测，收率为 89.4%。

3. Pd/TB-COF 催化加氢还原法制备苯佐卡因

（1）搭建实验装置。

Pd/TB-COF
催化加氢
还原法虚拟
仿真实验演示

（2）在反应釜中加入 3 mL 乙醇，0.064 g 对硝基苯甲酸乙酯和 0.0014 g 5% Pd/TB-COF。搅拌溶解，密封。

（3）进行氮气置换。

（4）进行氢气置换。

（5）调节氢气压力为 20 atm（2 MPa），40 ℃下反应 3 h。记录反应过程中压力、温度变化。

（6）反应完毕，停止加热、冷却、关闭进气开关、打开排气阀泄压。

（7）进行氮气置换。

（8）打开反应釜。

（9）取样，经高效液相色谱法（HPLC）检测，收率为 99.0%。

4. 催化氢转移法制备苯佐卡因

（1）搭建实验装置。

催化氢转移
法虚拟实验
实验演示

（2）称取 1.95 g 对硝基苯甲酸乙酯和 2.27 g 甲酸铵加入三口烧瓶，加入无水乙醇 30 mL。

(3) 设定反应温度为 25 ℃。开启搅拌。

(4) 称取 0.1 g 10％Pd/C，通过加料漏斗加入三口烧瓶中。

(5) 25 ℃下继续搅拌 1 h 后，用毛细管点样，进行薄层色谱法（TLC）分析（TLC 展开剂为石油醚∶乙酸乙酯＝4∶1）。

(6) 反应完毕，过滤除去固体，用 200 mL 乙醇洗涤滤渣。滤液用于下步后处理。

(7) 将滤液用旋转蒸发仪蒸干，得到 1.54 g 白色固体。该白色固体为苯佐卡因，收率为 93.3％。

V 实验结果

1. 收率

(1) Pd/C 催化加氢还原法所获得的苯佐卡因的收率为 89.4％。

(2) Pd/TB-COF 催化加氢还原法所获得的苯佐卡因的收率为 99.0％。

(3) 催化氢转移法所获得的苯佐卡因的收率为 93.3％。

2. 产品外观与熔点

A. 外观：_____；

B. 熔点：

　　理论值：88～90 ℃；

　　实测值：87～89 ℃。

3. 核磁共振氢谱

^{1}H NMR（300 MHz，CDCl$_3$）δ：1.3(3H，t)，4.1(2H，s)，4.3(2H，m)，6.6(2H，d)，7.8(2H，d)。

4. 实验结果分析

_____

_____

_____

_____

_____

_____

_____

_____。

VI 注意事项

1. 氢气钢瓶的颜色是深绿色，字体的颜色是红色。应保持氢气钢瓶漆色和字样鲜明。氢气钢瓶应储存于阴凉、通风的库房，库温不宜超过 30 ℃，远离火种、热源，防止阳光直射；氢气钢瓶应与氧气、压缩空气、卤素（氟、氯、溴）、氧化剂等分开存放，切忌混储混运；氢气钢瓶、氢化釜及其管道应定期进行安全检查，包括检查外观、定点测量壁厚、定时测量壁温和分析腐蚀介质成分，应采取氮气气封、对反应器内壁采取无损检测、内壁宏观检查等方法，重点检查焊缝区、堆焊层及螺栓、螺母垫圈和容器内外支承结构，必要时采取气密性或水压试验等措施以确保加氢反应器的使用安全。钢瓶发生氢脆现象与多种因素有关，控制氢脆现象最重要的措施应为限制钢种并控制所含杂质的种类和含量、控制钢的抗拉强度 $\sigma_b < 882$ MPa。

2. 安装氢化釜时，必须按照对角线原则拧紧螺母。这样做的主要原因是避免受力不均而引起爆炸。加氢反应器运行期间，作业人员应严格执行工艺操作规程，必须确保反应温度平稳和压力平稳。开、停工前应编制合理的开、停工方案，停工时增加适当脱氢过程，避免紧急泄压和降温。进行氢气置换时，严禁采用氢气直接置换空气。若氢气泄漏或爆炸，首先应立即切断气源。

3. 氮气置换的意义为：氮的化学性质不活泼，不容易与其他物质发生化学反应，采用氮气置换出管道内的空气，可避免氢气与空气中的氧气形成可燃性混合物，从而避免内燃或爆炸的发生。

VII 思考题

1. 将 0.043 g 苯佐卡因溶于 0.5 mL 氘代氯仿，采用 300 MHz 的核磁共振仪，测得的核磁共振氢谱如下图（标示了峰的化学位移和氢的编号），试解析苯佐卡因的核磁共振氢谱。

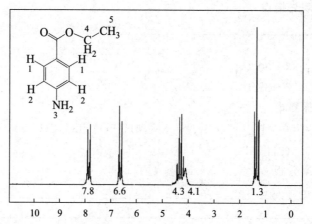

化学位移为 7.8 的峰对应的氢的编号为（　　　）；
化学位移为 6.6 的峰对应的氢的编号为（　　　）；
化学位移为 4.3 的峰对应的氢的编号为（　　　）；
化学位移为 4.1 的峰对应的氢的编号为（　　　）；
化学位移为 1.3 的峰对应的氢的编号为（　　　）。
2. 举例说明加氢还原法在药物合成中的应用。

（李雯）

Synthesis of Lidocaine Hydrochloride

Background

Lidocaine hydrochloride is a long-acting amide local anesthetic widely used in topical anesthesia, conduction anesthesia, infiltration anesthesia, and epidural anesthesia. Lidocaine hydrochloride is also a first-line medication for treating ventricular arrhythmias caused by acute and severe hemodynamic abnormalities. The chemical structure of Lidocaine hydrochloride is shown in Fig. 9-1.

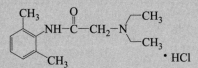

The mechanism of action of Lidocaine hydrochloride

Fig. 9-1　Chemical structure of Lidocaine hydrochloride

Ⅰ Purposes and Requirements

1. To understand the reaction principle for preparing the chloroacetyl chloride compounds.

2. To understand the principle of *N*-alkylation reaction.

3. To master the experimental operation of synthesis of Lidocaine hydrochloride.

4. To understand the mode of action of lidocaine hydrochloride and its target.

Ⅱ Principle of the Reaction

1. Physical data of the main reactants and product

Name	Structure CAS No.	Formula M. Wt	b. p. or m. p. / ℃	Solubility
2,6-Dimethylaniline	$C_8H_{11}N$ 270.80 87-62-7	$C_8H_{11}N$ 270.80	m. p. 216	Insoluble in water

Name	Structure CAS No.	Formula M. Wt	b. p. or m. p. / ℃	Solubility
Chloroacetyl chloride	[structure] 79-04-9	$C_2H_2Cl_2O$ 112.94	b. p. 105~106	React with water. Soluble in commonly used organic solvents
2-Chloro-N-(2,6-dimethylphenyl)acetamide	[structure] 1131-01-7	$C_{10}H_{12}ClNO$ 197.66	m. p. 150~151	Soluble in chloroform, DMSO, methanol; insoluble in water
Diethylamine	[structure] 109-89-7	$C_4H_{11}N$ 73.14	b. p. 56	Completely miscible with water
Sodium acetate	CH_3COONa 127-09-3	$C_2H_3O_2Na$ 82.03	m. p. >300	Easy to dissolve in water
Potassium carbonate	K_2CO_3 584-08-7	K_2CO_3 138.21	m. p. 891	Easy to dissolve in water
Sodium bisulfite	$NaHSO_3$ 7631-90-5	$NaHSO_3$ 104.06	m. p. 150~152	Easy to dissolve in water, slightly soluble in ethanol
Lidocaine	[structure] 137-58-6	$C_{14}H_{22}N_2O$ 234.34	m. p. 66~69	Almost insoluble in water
Lidocaine hydrochloride	[structure] 73-78-9	$C_{14}H_{23}ClN_2O$ 270.80	m. p. 80~82	36 g/L in water at 20 ℃

2. Synthetic route

The synthesis of lidocaine hydrochloride involves the acylation reaction of 2,6-dimethylaniline and chloroacetyl chloride to obtain the intermediate 2-chloro-N-(2,6-dimethylphenyl) acetamide, which is then subjected to N-alkylation and salt formation reactions to obtain the target compound.

Safety Tips: Chloroacetyl chloride has an irritating odor and must be used in a fume hood. It can burn the skin and irritate mucous membranes. When chloroacetyl chloride comes into contact with water, it undergoes a violent reaction and produces toxic gases.

3. Knowledge points

Chloroacetylation reaction, N-alkylation reaction, acid binding agent, antioxidant.

Ⅲ Experimental Equipments and Raw Materials

1. Experimental equipment

The chloroacetylation reaction apparatus is composed of a magnetic stirrer, an ice-water bath, a three-neck round-bottom flask, a spherical condenser tube, and a thermometer.

The N-alkylation reaction apparatus is composed of a magnetic stirrer, a three-neck round-bottom flask, and a thermometer.

The chloroacetylation reaction apparatus and the N-alkylation reaction apparatus

2. Raw materials

Name	Quantity	Quality	Use
2,6-Dimethylaniline	5 mL (0.04 mol)	CP	Reactant
Chloroacetyl chloride	3.5 mL (0.044 mol)	CP	Chloroacetylation reagent
Acetic acid	32 mL	CP	Solvent
Sodium acetate	14.5 g (0.175 mol)	CP	Acid binding agent
Diethylamine	90 mL (0.873 mol)	CP	Reactant
Sodium bisulfite	0.5 g	CP	Antioxidant
10% sodium hydroxide solution	10 mL	CP	Base
Acetone	20 mL	AR	Solvent
Concentrated hydrochloric acid	1.2 mL (0.014 mol)	CP	Acid
Activated carbon	0.2 g	—	Decolorizing agent
Water	125 mL	—	Solvent

Ⅳ Operations

1. Preparation of 2-chloro-N- (2,6-dimethylphenyl) acetamide

(1) Equip the chloroacetylation reaction apparatus.

(2) Place a 100 mL three-necked flask in an ice-water bath, add 3.5 mL of chloroacetyl chloride, 5 mL of 2,6-dimethylaniline, and 32 mL of acetic acid solution, stir well, and then add sodium acetate aqueous solution (a solution prepared by dissolving 14.5 g of sodium acetate in 125 mL of water).

(3) After reacting in an ice-water bath for 10 min, remove the ice-water bath and continue the reaction at room temperature for 0.5 h.

(4) Filter, wash the filter cake with an appropriate amount of water, dry

Experimental procedure of preparation of 2-chloro-N- (2,6-dimethylphenyl) acetamide

the obtained solid, weigh it, and obtain 7 g of product.

2. Preparation of lidocaine

(1) Equip the *N*-alkylation reaction apparatus.

(2) In a 100 mL dry three-necked flask, add 7 g of the intermediate obtained in the previous step, 90 mL of diethylamine and 0.5 g of sodium bisulfite. Stir and mix well.

(3) Slowly heat to 55 ℃, reflux for 1.5 h, TLC detect the reaction until completion.

(4) Remove the excess diethylamine from the filtrate by rotary evaporation, pour the residue into water. Heat up until the solid dissolves, cool down, and precipitate the solid.

(5) Filter, wash with water, and dry to obtain 3 g of off white product.

3. Preparation of lidocaine hydrochloride

(1) Equip the *N*-alkylation apparatus.

(2) Add 3 g of lidocaine prepared in the previous step and 20 mL of acetone to a 100 mL three-necked flask, stir well, and then add 1.2 mL of concentrated hydrochloric acid dropwise (lidocaine : concentrated hydrochloric acid＝1 g : 0.4 mL).

(3) After the dropwise addition is complete, heat to 45 ℃, add 0.2 g of activated carbon, then heat to 60 ℃, reflux for 10 min, hot filter, and get rid of the filter cake.

(4) Remove the solvent from the filtrate by rotary evaporation, add 6 mL of acetone to the residue, shake well, and place in an ice-water bath for 20 min to precipitate crystals.

(5) Filter, dry, and obtain the white product.

(6) Weigh, calculate yield, and measure melting point.

(7) Send the final product to the place where the teachers designated.

Ⅴ Experimental Results

1. Yield

(1) Calculate the theoretical production of lidocaine hydrochloride

$$\text{2,6-Dimethylaniline} \longrightarrow \text{Lidocaine Hydro}$$
$$M_w＝121.18 \text{ g/mol} \longrightarrow M_w＝270.80 \text{ g/mol}$$
$$0.04 \text{ mol} \longrightarrow 0.04 \text{ mol}$$
$$\text{Theoretical production}＝0.04 \text{ mol}\times270.80 \text{ g/mol}＝10.83 \text{ g}$$

(2) Calculate the percent yield of lidocaine hydrochloride

$$\text{Yield}＝\frac{\text{Practical production}}{\text{Theoretical production}}\times100\%＝\frac{(\quad\quad)}{10.83 \text{ g}}\times100\%＝(\quad\quad)\%$$

2. Appearance and melting point of product

A. Appearance： _____ ;

B. m. p. :

    Theoretical value：80～82 ℃

    Practical value： _____ .

3. Analysis of experimental results

_____

_____

_____

_____

_____

_____ .

Ⅵ Notes

1. To avoid the generation of by-products, the reaction should be slowly heated up.

2. The preparation step of lidocaine involves adding sodium bisulfite as an antioxidant.

3. During the salt formation reaction, the pH $= 4$ is more suitable for the system, and attention should be paid to the appropriate amount of hydrochloric acid added.

4. In this experiment, the preparation of lidocaine and lidocaine hydrochloride proceed from the previous step, and the amount of each reagent used needs to be calculated proportionally before use.

Ⅶ Determination of Product Content

Chromatographic conditions: using octadecylsilane bonded silica gel as the filler. Use phosphate buffer solution (take 1.3 mL of 1 mol/L sodium dihydrogen phosphate solution and 32.5 mL of 0.5 mol/L disodium hydrogen phosphate solution, dilute with water to 1000 mL, shake well)-acetonitrile (50 : 50) (adjust pH to 8.0 with phosphoric acid) as the mobile phase. The detection wavelength is 254 nm. The injection volume is 20 μL.

Measurement method: High-performance liquid chromatography method. Accurately weigh the test sample and reference solution, inject them separately into the liquid chromatograph, and record the chromatogram. Calculate the peak area using the external standard method and multiply the result by 1.156. (《Chinese Pharmacopoeia》 2020 Edition)

Ⅷ Discussion Questions

1. Why can the reaction be carried out in acetic acid/sodium acetate buffer when preparing 2-chloro-N-(2,6-dimethylphenyl) acetamide?

2. Why can chloroacetyl chloride react with 2,6-dimethylaniline and diethylamine successively?

(By Wen Li)

背景知识

盐酸利多卡因（Lidocaine hydrochloride）是一种长效的酰胺类局部麻醉药物，广泛用于表面麻醉、传导麻醉、浸润麻醉及硬膜外麻醉。盐酸利多卡因也是治疗急性和严重血流动力学异常引起的室性心律失常的一线药物。盐酸利多卡因的化学结构如图 9-1 所示。

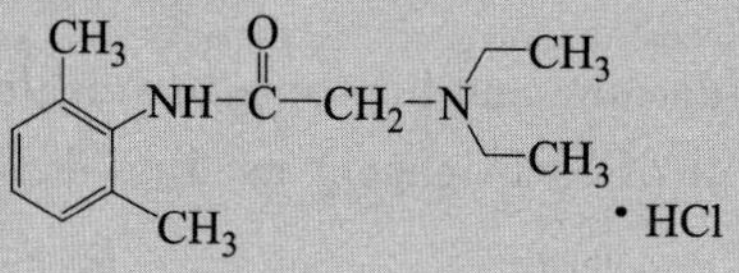

图 9-1　盐酸利多卡因的化学结构

盐酸利多卡因的作用机制

I　目的与要求

1. 理解制备氯乙酰氯化合物的反应原理。
2. 理解 N-烷基化反应的原理。
3. 掌握盐酸利多卡因合成的实验操作。
4. 了解盐酸利多卡因与靶标的作用方式。

II　实验原理

1. 主要反应物和产物的物理常数

名称	结构式 CAS 号	分子式 分子量	沸点或 熔点/℃	溶解性
2,6-二甲基苯胺	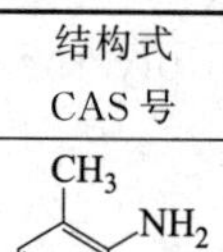 87-62-7	$C_8H_{11}N$ 270.80	m. p. 216	不溶于水
氯乙酰氯	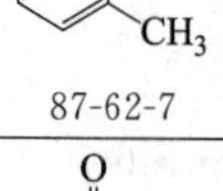 79-04-9	$C_2H_2Cl_2O$ 112.94	b. p. 105～106	和水反应。可溶于常用有机溶剂
2-氯-N-(2,6-二甲苯基) 乙酰胺	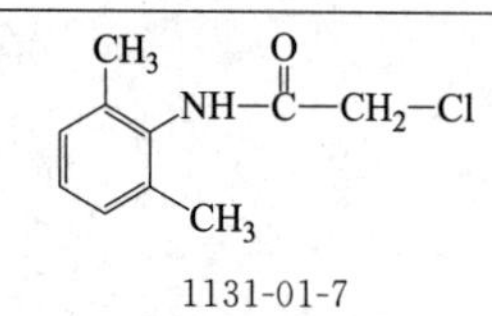 1131-01-7	$C_{10}H_{12}ClNO$ 197.66	m. p. 150～151	可溶于氯仿、DMSO、甲醇，不溶于水

名称	结构式 CAS 号	分子式 分子量	沸点或 熔点/℃	溶解性
二乙胺	HN（CH₃）₂ 109-89-7	$C_4H_{11}N$ 73.14	b. p. 56	和水完全混溶
醋酸钠	CH_3COONa 127-09-3	$C_2H_3NaO_2$ 82.03	m. p. ＞300	易溶于水
碳酸钾	K_2CO_3 584-08-7	K_2CO_3 138.21	m. p. 891	易溶于水
亚硫酸氢钠	$NaHSO_3$ 7631-90-5	$NaHSO_3$ 104.06	m. p. 150～152	易溶于水,微溶于乙醇
利多卡因	137-58-6	$C_{14}H_{22}N_2O$ 234.34	m. p. 66～69	几乎不溶于水
盐酸利多卡因	73-78-9	$C_{14}H_{23}ClN_2O$ 270.80	m. p. 80～82	20 ℃水中溶解度为 36 g/L

2. 合成路线

盐酸利多卡因的合成是以 2,6-二甲基苯胺和氯乙酰氯为原料，经酰化反应制得中间体 2-氯-N-(2,6-二甲苯基) 乙酰胺，然后再经 N-烷基化和成盐反应制得目标化合物。

安全提示：氯乙酰氯有刺激性气味，会灼伤皮肤，刺激黏膜，必须在通风橱中使用。氯乙酰氯遇水剧烈反应，并且产生有毒气体。

3. 知识点

氯乙酰化反应，N-烷基化反应，缚酸剂，抗氧剂。

Ⅲ 实验装置和原料

1. 实验装置

酰化反应装置由磁力搅拌器、冰水浴、三口烧瓶、回流冷凝管和温度计组成。

酰化反应装置和烷基化反应装置

烷基化反应装置由磁力搅拌器、三口烧瓶和温度计组成。

2. 原料

名称	用量	规格	用途
2,6-二甲基苯胺	5 mL(0.04 mol)	化学纯	反应物
氯乙酰氯	3.5 mL(0.044 mol)	化学纯	氯乙酰化试剂
醋酸	32 mL	化学纯	溶剂
醋酸钠	14.5 g(0.175 mol)	化学纯	缚酸剂
二乙胺	90 mL(0.873 mol)	化学纯	反应物
亚硫酸氢钠	0.5 g	化学纯	抗氧剂
10%氢氧化钠溶液	10 mL	化学纯	碱
丙酮	20 mL	分析纯	溶剂
浓盐酸	1.2 mL(0.014 mol)	化学纯	酸
活性炭	0.2 g	—	脱色剂
水	125 mL	—	溶剂

IV 实验操作

1. 2-氯-N-(2,6-二甲苯基) 乙酰胺的制备

(1) 搭建酰化反应装置。

(2) 将干燥的 100 mL 三口烧瓶置于冰水浴中，加入 3.5 mL 氯乙酰氯、5 mL 2,6-二甲基苯胺和 32 mL 醋酸溶液，搅拌均匀后，加入醋酸钠水溶液（14.5 g 醋酸钠溶于 125 mL 水制得的溶液）。

(3) 冰水浴反应 10 min 后，撤去冰水浴，常温条件下继续反应 0.5 h。

(4) 过滤，滤饼用适量水洗涤，将所得固体干燥，称重，得到产物 7 g。

2. 利多卡因的制备

(1) 搭建烷基化反应装置。

(2) 向干燥的 100 mL 三口烧瓶中加入 7 g 上步制得的中间体、90 mL 二乙胺、0.5 g 亚硫酸氢钠，搅拌均匀。

(3) 缓慢加热至 55 ℃，回流 1.5 h，TLC 检测反应至完成反应。

(4) 将滤液旋蒸除去过量的二乙胺，残余物倒入水中，升温至固体溶解，冷却，析出固体。

(5) 过滤，水洗，干燥，得到米白色产物 3 g。

3. 盐酸利多卡因的制备

(1) 搭建烷基化反应装置。

(2) 向 100 mL 三口烧瓶中加入 3 g 上步制得的利多卡因、20 mL 丙酮，搅拌均匀后，滴加 1.2 mL 浓盐酸（利多卡因∶浓盐酸＝1 g∶0.4 mL）。

(3) 滴加完毕，升温至 45 ℃，加入 0.2 g 活性炭，然后加热至 60 ℃，回流 10 min，热过滤，弃去滤饼。

(4) 将滤液旋蒸除去溶剂，在残留物中加入 6 mL 丙酮，摇匀后，置于冰水浴中 20 min，析出晶体。

(5) 过滤，干燥，得到白色产物。

(6) 称重，计算收率，测熔点。

(7) 将产物送到指导教师指定的产品回收处。

V 实验结果

1. 收率

(1) 计算盐酸利多卡因的理论产量。

$$2,6\text{-二甲基苯胺}\text{————}盐酸利多卡因$$

$$M_w=121.18 \text{ g/mol} \text{————} M_w=270.80 \text{ g/mol}$$

$$0.04 \text{ mol} \text{————} 0.04 \text{ mol}$$

理论产量 $=0.04 \text{ mol} \times 270.80 \text{ g/mol}=10.83 \text{ g}$

(2) 计算盐酸利多卡因的收率

$$收率=\frac{产品实际产量}{产品理论产量}\times 100\%=\frac{(\quad)}{10.83 \text{ g}}\times 100\%=(\qquad)\%$$

2. 产品外观与熔点

A. 外观：_____；

B. 熔点：

理论值：80~82 ℃；

实测值：_____。

3. 实验结果分析

_____
_____
_____
_____
_____
_____
_____。

VI 注意事项

1. 为了避免副产物的生成，反应要缓慢升温。

2. 利多卡因的制备步骤中，加入的亚硫酸氢钠为抗氧剂。

3. 成盐反应时，体系 pH = 4 较为合适，应注意加入盐酸的量应适宜。

4. 本实验中，利多卡因和盐酸利多卡因的制备是接着上一步反应进行的，所用试剂的量需要按照比例计算后使用。

VII 产物的含量测定

色谱条件：以十八烷基硅烷键合硅胶为填充剂；以磷酸盐缓冲液（取 1 mol/L 磷酸二氢钠溶液 1.3 mL 与 0.5 mol/L 磷酸氢二钠溶液 32.5 mL，用水稀释至 1000 mL，摇匀)-乙腈（50∶50）（用磷酸调节 pH 值至 8.0）为流动相；检测波长为 254 nm；进样体积 20 μL。

测定法：高效液相色谱法。精密称定供试品与对照品溶液，分别注入液相色谱仪，记录色谱图。按照外标法以峰面积计算，并将结果乘以 1.156。(《中华人

民共和国药典（2020 年版)》》

Ⅷ 思考题

1. 制备 2-氯-*N*-(2,6-二甲苯基）乙酰胺时，为什么反应可以在醋酸/醋酸钠缓冲液中进行？

2. 为什么氯乙酰氯可以先后和 2,6-二甲基苯胺、二乙胺反应？

（李雯）

Experiment 10

Synthesis of Dyclonine Hydrochloride

Background

Dyclonine hydrochloride, also named dacronin, is an aminoketone local anesthetic developed by Astrazeneca Company. It has been used in China since 2002. This product has the advantages of strong mucosal penetration, rapid response and lasting effect. Clinically, it is used for analgesia of burns and abrasions, and for preparation before endoscopy such as laryngoscope, tracheoscope and cystoscopy. The chemical structure of Dyclonine hydrochloride is shown in Fig. 10-1.

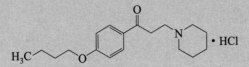

The mechanism of action of Dyclonine hydrochloride

Fig. 10-1   Structure of Dyclonine hydrochloride

Ⅰ Purposes and Requirements

1. To master the principle and operation requirements of the O-alkylation reaction, Mannich reaction.

2. To master the method of recrystallization purification.

3. To get familiar with experimental operations of thin-layer chromatography.

4. To understand the interaction between dyclonine hydrochloride and target.

Ⅱ Principle of the Reaction

1. Physical data of the main reactants and product

Name	Structure CAS No.	Formula M. Wt	b. p. or m. p. /℃	Solubility
p-Hydroxyaceto-phenone	99-93-4	$C_8H_8O_2$ 136. 15	m. p. 107~111	Well soluble in hot water, methanol, ethanol, ether, acetone, and benzene. Insoluble in petroleum ether

Name	Structure CAS No.	Formula M. Wt	b. p. or m. p. /℃	Solubility
1-(4-Butoxyphenyl) ethanone	n-C$_4$H$_9^*$O—⟨⟩—COCH$_3$ 5736-89-0	C$_{12}$H$_{16}$O$_2$ 192.25	m. p. 25～27	Soluble in methanol
Dyclonine hydrochloride	n-C$_4$H$_9^*$O—⟨⟩—CO—CH$_2$—N⟨piperidine⟩ · HCl 586-60-7	C$_{18}$H$_{27}$NO$_2$ 289.41	m. p. 175～176	Well soluble in water, soluble in chloroform, acetone and methanol
1-Bromobutane	H$_3$C———Br 109-65-9	C$_4$H$_9$Br 137.03	b. p. 101.6	Insoluble in water, soluble in alcohol, ether, benzene, carbon tetrachloride and other organic solvents
Potassium carbonate	K$_2$CO$_3$ 584-08-7	K$_2$CO$_3$ 138.21	m. p. 891	Well soluble in water
N, N-Dimethylformamide	HC(=O)—N(CH$_3$)CH$_3$ 68-12-2	C$_3$H$_7$NO 73.09	b. p. 153	Miscible in most organic solvents and water
Paraformaldehyde	(HCHO)$_n$ 30525-89-4	(CH$_2$O)$_n$ (30)$_n$	m. p. 120～170	Soluble in dilute alkali and acid solution, more soluble in hot water, insoluble in ethanol and ether
Piperidine hydrochloride	⟨⟩NH · HCl 6091-44-7	C$_5$H$_{12}$ClN 121.61	m. p. 245～248	Well soluble in water and ethanol
Hydrochloric acid	HCl 7647-01-0	HCl 36.5	b. p. 48(38% solutinon)	Aqueous solution
Anhydrous sodium sulfate	Na$_2$SO$_4$ 7757-82-6	Na$_2$SO$_4$ 142.04	m. p. 884	Soluble in water

* n-C$_4$H$_9$＝CH$_3$CH$_2$CH$_2$CH$_2$

2. Synthetic route

p-Hydroxyacetophenone $\xrightarrow{n\text{-C}_4\text{H}_9\text{Br/ K}_2\text{CO}_3}$ 1-(4-Butoxyphenyl)ethanone

$\xrightarrow{\text{(HCHO)}_n,\ \text{⟨⟩NH · HCl}}$ Dyclonine hydrochloride

1-(4-Butoxyphenyl) ethanone is obtained by O-alkylation from p-hydroxyacetophenone and n-bromobutane. Then, 1-(4-butoxyphenyl) ethanone, polyformaldehyde, and piperidine hydrochloride will undergo mannich condensation to form dyclonine hydrochloride.

Safety Tips: A small amount of concentrated hydrochloric acid is used in the experiment. Concentrated hydrochloric acid may corrode metals, cause serious skin burns and eye damage, and may cause respiratory irritation. Concentrated hydrochloric acid should be accessed in a fume hood, wearing a lab coat and protective gloves. If the skin (or hair) is contaminated with concentrated hydrochloric acid, immediately remove all clothing contaminated with concentrated hydrochloric acid, wash the skin with plenty of water/shower for more than 15 minutes, and seek medical attention; If it enters the eyes, carefully rinse with water for at least 15 minutes (including under the eyelids) and seek medical attention.

3. Knowledge points
O-alkylation reaction, Mannich reaction, thin-layer chromatography.

Ⅲ Experimental Equipments and Raw Materials

1. Experimental equipment
The O-alkylation reaction apparatus is composed of a three-neck round-bottom flask, a spherical condenser tube, a magnetic stirrer, and a thermometer.

The O-alkylation reaction apparatus

2. Raw materials

Synthetic product	Raw materials			
	Name	Quantity	Quality	Use
1-(4-Butoxyphenyl) ethanone	p-Hydroxyacetophenone	6.8 g (0.05 mol)	CP	Reactant
	1-Bromobutane	5.4 mL (0.05 mol)	CP	Reactant
	Potassium carbonate	13.8 g (0.10 mol)	CP	Reactant
	N,N-Dimethylformamide	50 mL	CP	Solvent
	Distilled water	280 mL	—	Solvent
	Anhydrous sodium sulfate	3 g	CP	Dehydrant
	Petroleum ether(PE)	10 mL	AR	TLC developer
	Ethyl acetate(EA)	150 mL	AR	Extractant and TLC developer
Dyclonine hydrochloride	1-(4-Butoxyphenyl)ethanone	8.7 g (0.045 mol)	Product prepared	Reactant
	Paraformaldehyde	2.7 g (0.09 mol)	CP	Reactant
	Piperidine hydrochloride	7.3 g (0.06 mol)	CP	Reactant
	Concentrated hydrochloric acid	0.6 mL	CP	Catalytic agent
	Isopropyl alcohol	50 mL	CP	Solvent
	Distilled water	Appropriate amount	—	Solvent
	Petroleum ether	Appropriate amount	AR	TLC developer
	Ethyl acetate	30 mL	AR	TLC developer

Experimental procedure of preparation of 1-(4-butoxyphenyl) ethanone

Ⅳ Operations

1. Preparation of 1-(4-butoxyphenyl) ethanone

(1) Equip the reaction apparatus.

(2) Add 6.8 g p-hydroxyacetophenone, 50 mL N,N-dimethylformamide and 13.8 g anhydrous potassium carbonate into a 100 mL three-necked round-bottom flask, stir and mix well.

(3) Add 5.4 mL 1-bromobutane. Keep stirring, slowly heat to 85 ℃ and react for 1 h. The endpoint of the reaction can be monitored by thin-layer chromatography. (TLC developing solvent is PE∶EA=3∶1)

(4) Then, transfer the reaction solution to a 100 mL separatory funnel, add 100 mL of water, and shake well.

(5) Extract the above solution with 50 mL of ethyl acetate 3 times (50 mL×3), combine the ethyl acetate solutions.

(6) Wash the obtained ethyl acetate solution with 30 mL water 6 times (30 mL×6).

(7) Dry the ethyl acetate solution with anhydrous sodium sulfate.

(8) Remove the solvent by rotary evaporation to obtain colorless oily substance. Weigh the oil and calculate the yield.

2. Preparation of dyclonine hydrochloride

Experimental procedure of preparation of dyclonine hydrochloride

(1) Equip the reaction apparatus.

(2) Add 8.7 g 1-(4-butoxyphenyl) ethanone, 2.7 g paraformaldehyde, 7.3 g piperidine hydrochloride, and 50 mL isopropyl alcohol into a 100 mL three-necked round-bottom flask, stir and mix well. Add 0.6 mL concentrated hydrochloric acid to the flask.

(3) Keep stirring, slowly heat to 85 ℃ and reflux for 2.5 h. The endpoint of the reaction can be monitored by thin-layer chromatography (TLC developing solvent is PE∶EA=3∶1). Cool to room temperature.

(4) Transfer the hot mixture to the 100 mL beaker, and then cool it in an ice bath to precipitate the solids.

(5) Filter, dry the obtained solid, weigh it, and obtain 7 g of crude product.

(6) Equip the reaction apparatus.

(7) In a 100 mL three-neck round-bottom flask, the crude product was recrystallized using ethanol-water (1∶9). The ratio is crude product∶ethanol-water=1 g∶8 mL.

(8) The mixture is heated and dissolved, cooled to room temperature. The solid is precipitated.

(9) Filter and wash the filter cake with a small amount of cold ethanol to obtain the refined product of Dyclonine hydrochloride.

(10) Dry the product, weigh it, calculate the yield, and measure the melting point.

(11) Send the final product to the place where the teachers designated.

V Experimental Results

1. Yield

(1) Calculate the theoretical production of dyclonine hydrochloride

p-Hydroxyacetophenone —————— Dyclonine hydrochloride

$M_w = 136.15$ g/mol —————— $M_w = 289.41$ g/mol

0.05 mol —————— 0.05 mol

Theoretical production $= 0.05$ mol $\times 289.41$ g/mol $= 14.47$ g

(2) Calculate the percent yield of dyclonine hydrochloride

$$\text{Yield} = \frac{\text{Practical production}}{\text{Theoretical production}} \times 100\% = \frac{(\quad)}{14.47 \text{ g}} \times 100\% = (\quad)\%$$

2. Appearance and melting point of product

A. Appearance: _____ ;

B. m. p. :

Theoretical value: $175 \sim 176$ ℃

Practical value: _____ .

3. Analysis of experimental results

_____

_____

_____

_____

_____

_____

_____ .

VI Notes

1. Usually, in order to promote reaction, Mannich reaction needs to use an oil-water separator to remove water from the reaction system. After multiple experimental studies, the preparation of dyclonine hydrochloride can still obtain a higher yield when using the isopropyl alcohol reflux method without oil-water separator. The reaction operation is simpler.

2. In this experimental, the preparation of dyclonine hydrochloride proceeded from the previous reaction. So, the amount of each reagent used should be calculated proportionally.

VII Determination of Product Content

Chromatographic conditions: Triethylsilane chemically bonded fully porous silica gel microspheres were used as fillers. Dissolve 0.20 g of potassium dihydrogen phosphate and 0.45 mL of n-heptamine in approximately 350 mL of water, adjust the pH to 3.0 with phosphoric acid, dilute to 400 mL with water, add 600 mL of acetonitrile, and mix to obtain the mobile phase. The flow rate is 1.2 mL/min. The detection wavelength is 254 nm. The injection volume is 20 μL.

Measurement method: High-performance liquid chromatography method. Precisely weigh the test sample and reference solution, inject them into the liquid chromatograph separately, and record the chromatogram. Calculate based on peak area using the external standard method. (USP-NF2024 edition of the United States Pharmacopeia)

Ⅷ Discussion Questions

1. In terms of structure, why does p-hydroxyacetophenone dissolve in potassium carbonate aqueous solution?

2. In terms of structure, explain the reaction mechanism of Mannich condensation to dyclonine hydrochloride.

(By Kai Sun)

实验十

盐酸达克罗宁的合成

背景知识

盐酸达克罗宁（Dyclonine Hydrochloride）是 Astrazeneca 公司开发的氨基酮类局部麻醉药物，2002 年在我国开始应用。该品具有黏膜穿透力强、显效快，作用持久等优点，临床用于火伤、擦伤的镇痛，以及喉镜、气管镜、膀胱镜等内窥镜检查前的准备，其化学结构见图 10-1。

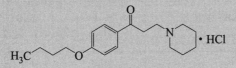

图 10-1 盐酸达克罗宁的化学结构

盐酸达克罗宁
的作用机制

I 目的与要求

1. 掌握 *O*-烷基化反应、Mannich 反应的原理和操作要求。
2. 掌握重结晶纯化的原理。
3. 熟悉薄层色谱法的实验操作。
4. 了解盐酸达克罗宁与靶标的作用方式。

II 实验原理

1. 主要反应物和产物的物理常数

名称	结构式 CAS 号	分子式 分子量	沸点或 熔点/℃	溶解度
对羟基苯乙酮	(见结构式) 99-93-4	$C_8H_8O_2$ 136.15	m. p. 107～111	易溶于热水、甲醇、乙醇、乙醚、丙酮、苯,难溶于石油醚
对正丁氧基苯乙酮	(见结构式) 5736-89-0	$C_{12}H_{16}O_2$ 192.25	m. p. 25～27	溶于甲醇

名称	结构式 CAS 号	分子式 分子量	沸点或 熔点/℃	溶解度
盐酸达克罗宁	$n\text{-}C_4H_9^*O$——苯环——$C(=O)CH_2CH_2N$(哌啶)$\cdot HCl$ 586-60-7	$C_{18}H_{27}NO_2$ 289.41	m. p. 175～176	易溶于水,溶于氯仿、丙酮和甲醇
正溴丁烷	H_3C——Br 109-65-9	C_4H_9Br 137.03	b. p. 101.6	不溶于水,能溶于醇、醚、苯、四氯化碳等有机溶剂
碳酸钾	K_2CO_3 584-08-7	K_2CO_3 138.21	m. p. 891	易溶于水
N,N-二甲基甲酰胺	$HC(=O)N(CH_3)_2$ 68-12-2	C_3H_7NO 73.09	b. p. 153	与水混溶,可混溶于多数有机溶剂
多聚甲醛	$(HCHO)_n$ 30525-89-4	$(CH_2O)_n$ $(30)_n$	m. p. 120～170	溶于稀碱和稀酸溶液,较易溶于热水,不溶于醇和醚
哌啶盐酸盐	$NH\cdot HCl$(哌啶) 6091-44-7	$C_5H_{12}ClN$ 121.61	m. p. 245～248	易溶于水和乙醇
盐酸	HCl 7647-01-0	HCl 36.5	b. p. 48(38%溶液)	水溶液
无水硫酸钠	Na_2SO_4 7757-82-6	Na_2SO_4 142.04	m. p. 884	溶于水

* $n\text{-}C_4H_9 = CH_3CH_2CH_2CH_2$

2. 合成路线

对羟基苯乙酮 $\xrightarrow{n\text{-}C_4H_9Br/\ K_2CO_3}$ 对正丁氧基苯乙酮

$\xrightarrow[\text{哌啶 } NH\cdot HCl]{(HCHO)_n,}$ 盐酸达克罗宁

对羟基苯乙酮与正溴丁烷发生 O-烷基化反应生成对正丁氧基苯乙酮,然后与多聚甲醛和盐酸哌啶发生 Mannich 缩合生成盐酸达克罗宁。

安全提示:实验中用到少量浓盐酸。浓盐酸具有强腐蚀性,可导致皮肤严重灼伤,接触眼睛可能造成永久性损伤。此外,其挥发性气体可能刺激呼吸道,导

致咳嗽、呼吸困难。因此，操作时务必在通风橱内进行，并佩戴防护手套和护目镜。如皮肤（或头发）沾染浓盐酸，应立即脱掉所有沾染浓盐酸的衣服，用大量水清洗皮肤/淋浴 15 分钟以上并就医；如进入眼睛，应用水小心冲洗 15 分钟以上（包括眼皮下面）并就医。

O-烷基化
反应装置

3. 知识点

O-烷基化反应，Mannich 反应，薄层色谱法。

Ⅲ 实验装置和原料

1. 实验装置

O-烷基化反应装置由三口烧瓶，回流冷凝管，磁力搅拌器和温度计组成。

2. 原料

合成产物	原料			
	名称	用量	试剂级别	用途
对正丁氧基苯乙酮	对羟基苯乙酮	6.8 g(0.05 mol)	化学纯	反应物
	正溴丁烷	5.4 mL(0.05 mol)	化学纯	反应物
	碳酸钾	13.8 g(0.10 mol)	化学纯	反应物
	N,N-二甲基甲酰胺	50 mL	化学纯	溶剂
	蒸馏水	280 mL	—	溶剂
	无水硫酸钠	3 g	化学纯	除水剂
	石油醚	10 mL	分析纯	薄层色谱法展开剂
	乙酸乙酯	150 mL	分析纯	萃取剂和薄层色谱法展开剂
盐酸达克罗宁	对正丁氧基苯乙酮	8.7 g(0.045 mol)	自制	反应物
	多聚甲醛	2.7 g(0.09 mol)	化学纯	反应物
	哌啶盐酸盐	7.3 g(0.06 mol)	化学纯	反应物
	浓盐酸	0.6 mL	化学纯	催化剂
	异丙醇	50 mL	化学纯	溶剂
	蒸馏水	适量	—	溶剂
	石油醚	适量	分析纯	薄层色谱法展开剂
	乙酸乙酯	30 mL	分析纯	薄层色谱法展开剂

Ⅳ 实验操作

1. 对正丁氧基苯乙酮的合成

（1）搭建反应装置。

（2）在 100 mL 三口烧瓶中，加入 6.8 g 对羟基苯乙酮，50 mL N,N-二甲基甲酰胺，13.8 g 碳酸钾，搅拌均匀。

（3）加入 5.4 mL 正溴丁烷，搅拌，缓慢升温至 85 ℃反应 1 h。反应终点可用薄层色谱法（TLC）进行检测（TLC 展开剂为石油醚∶乙酸乙酯＝3∶1）。冷却至室温。

（4）将反应液转移至 100 mL 分液漏斗中，加入 100 mL 水，摇匀。

（5）用 50 mL 乙酸乙酯萃取以上溶液 3 次（50 mL×3），合并乙酸乙酯萃取液。

（6）用 30 mL 水洗涤以上溶液 6 次（30 mL×6）。

（7）无水硫酸钠干燥乙酸乙酯萃取液。

（8）旋蒸除去溶剂后获得无色油状物。称重，计算收率。

2. 盐酸达克罗宁的合成

（1）搭建反应装置。

（2）在 100 mL 三口烧瓶中，加入 8.7 g 对正丁氧基苯乙酮，2.7 g 多聚甲醛，7.3 g 盐酸哌啶，50 mL 异丙醇，搅拌均匀。加入 0.6 mL 浓盐酸。

（3）搅拌，缓慢升温至 85 ℃，回流反应 2.5 h。反应终点可用薄层色谱法（TLC）进行检测（TLC 展开剂为石油醚：乙酸乙酯＝3：1）。冷却至室温。

（4）将反应液趁热转移至 100 mL 烧杯中，冰浴冷却析晶。

（5）抽滤，干燥所得到的固体，称重，获得 7 g 粗品。

（6）搭建反应装置。

（7）在 100 mL 三口烧瓶中，粗品用乙醇-水（1：9）重结晶，比例为粗品：乙醇-水＝1 g：8 mL。

（8）加热溶解后，冷却至室温，析出固体。

（9）抽滤，少量冷乙醇洗涤滤饼，得到盐酸达克罗宁精制品。

（10）干燥产品，称重，计算收率，测熔点。

（11）将产物送到指导教师指定的产品回收处。

V 实验结果

1. 收率

（1）计算盐酸达克罗宁的理论产量

$$对羟基苯乙酮————盐酸达克罗宁$$
$$M_w=136.15\ g/mol————M_w=289.41\ g/mol$$
$$0.05\ mol————0.05\ mol$$
$$理论产量＝0.05\ mol×289.41\ g/mol＝14.47\ g$$

（2）计算盐酸达克罗宁的收率

$$收率＝\frac{产品实际产量}{产品理论产量}×100\%＝\frac{(\qquad)}{14.47\ g}×100\%＝(\qquad)\%$$

2. 产品外观与熔点

A. 外观：＿＿＿＿＿＿＿＿＿＿＿＿＿＿＿＿＿＿＿＿＿＿＿；

B. 熔点：

理论值：175～176 ℃；

实测值：＿＿＿＿＿＿＿＿＿＿＿＿＿＿＿＿＿。

3. 实验结果分析

＿＿＿

＿＿＿

＿＿＿

＿＿＿

＿＿＿

＿＿。

Ⅵ 注意事项

1. 通常情况下，Mannich 反应需要采用油水分离器将水从反应体系中除去以促进反应进行，经反复探索，盐酸达克罗宁的制备，采用乙醇回流的方法，不必采用分水装置，依然可以得到较高收率，反应操作更为简便。

2. 本实验中，盐酸达克罗宁的合成是接着上一步反应进行的，所用试剂的量需要按照比例计算后使用。

Ⅶ 产物的含量测定

色谱条件：以三乙基硅烷化学键合全多孔硅胶微球为填充剂；将 0.20 g 磷酸二氢钾和 0.45 mL 正庚胺溶解在约 350 mL 水中，用磷酸调节 pH 至 3.0，用水稀释至 400 mL，加入 600 mL 乙腈，混合得到流动相；流速为 1.2 mL/min；检测波长为 254 nm；进样体积 20 μL。

测定法：采用高效液相色谱法。精密称定供试品与对照品溶液，分别注入液相色谱仪，记录色谱图。按照外标法以峰面积计算。（美国药典 USP-NF2024 版）

Ⅷ 思考题

1. 用结构式表示，为什么对羟基苯乙酮溶于碳酸钾水溶液？
2. 用结构式表示，Mannich 缩合生成盐酸达克罗宁的反应机理。

（孙凯）

Experiment 11

Synthesis of Nitrendipine

Background

Nitrendipine, a second-generation 1,4-dihydropyridine calcium channel blocker, was initially introduced in Germany in 1985 for treatment of hypertension, congestive heart failure, and angina pectoris associated with hypertension (Fig. 11-1). It selectively targets L-type calcium channels in vascular smooth muscle to inhibit transmembrane calcium ion influx between vascular smooth muscle and myocardium. With a higher affinity for blood vessels than myocardium, it exhibits a stronger selective effect on coronary arteries while reducing myocardial oxygen consumption and providing protective effects on ischemic myocardium. Additionally, it effectively lowers blood pressure by decreasing total peripheral resistance.

The mechanism of action of Nitrendipine

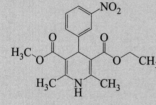

Fig. 11-1 Structure of Nitrendipine

Ⅰ Purposes and Requirements

1. To master the synthesis operation of nitrendipine.

2. To familiar with the fundamental principles of Knoevenagel condensation reaction and Michael addition reaction.

3. To understand the main sources of impurities in nitrendipine.

Ⅱ Principle of the Reaction

1. Physical data of the main reactants and product

Name	Structure CAS No.	Formula M. Wt	b. p. or m. p. /℃	Solubility
3-Nitrobenzaldehyde	O₂N—CHO 99-61-6	$C_7H_5NO_3$ 151.12	m. p. 56~59	1.6 mg/mL in water(20 ℃), well soluble in commonly used organic solvents

Name	Structure CAS No.	Formula M. Wt	b. p. or m. p. /℃	Solubility
Ethyl acetoacetate	H_3C ⋯ O ⋯ CH_3 141-97-9	$C_6H_{10}O_3$ 130. 14	b. p. 180. 8	2. 86 g/100 mL in water(20 ℃), well soluble in commonly used organic solvents
Acetic anhydride	H_3C ⋯ O ⋯ CH_3 108-24-7	$C_4H_6O_3$ 102. 09	b. p. 140	Slowly dissolves in water to form acetic acid, well soluble in chloroform and diethyl ether
Methyl 3-aminocrotonate	NH_2 O H_3C ⋯ O ⋯ CH_3 14205-39-1	$C_5H_9NO_2$ 115. 13	m. p. 81~83	Well soluble in commonly used organic solvents
Ethyl 3-nitrobenzylidene-acetoacetate	NO_2 ... O ⋯ CH_3 H_3C O 39562-16-8	$C_{13}H_{13}NO_5$ 263. 25	m. p. 162~164	Insoluble in water, well soluble in acetone, dichloromethane, and chloroform. Slightly soluble in methanol and ethanol
Nitrendipine	NO_2 ... H_3C O ⋯ O ⋯ CH_3 H_3C N CH_3 H 39562-70-4	$C_{18}H_{20}N_2O_6$ 360. 36	m. p. 169~171	Insoluble in water, well soluble in acetone, dichloromethane, and chloroform. Slightly soluble in methanol and ethanol

2. Synthetic route

3-Nitrobenzaldehyde + Ethyl acetoacetate $\xrightarrow{(CH_3CO)_2O, H_2SO_4}$ Ethyl 3-Nitrobenzylideneacetoacetate

$\xrightarrow{HCl, C_2H_5OH}$ Nitrendipine

The synthesis of nitrendipine is based on 3-nitrobenzaldehyde and ethyl acetoacetate as raw materials. The intermediate is obtained through the Knoevenagel condensation reaction in the presence of acetic anhydride and concentrated sulfuric acid, and then the target compound is obtained through Michael addition and cyclization reaction.

During the cyclization reaction, under acidic conditions at 70 ℃, the dihydro-pyridine ring is prone to undergo oxidation reactions to produce pyridine compounds. In addition, at 70 ℃ and acidic conditions, ester exchange reactions are prone to occur, generating small amounts of dimethyl esters and diethyl esters.

Pyridine compound   Dimethyl esters   Diethyl esters

Safety Tips: Acetic anhydride and concentrated hydrochloric acid can cause skin burns and emit an irritating odor; therefore, it is recommended to handle them in a fume hood. In the event that acetic anhydride and concentrated hydrochloric come into contact with the skin, immediate rinsing with abundant water is advised. If there is exposure to concentrated sulfuric acid on the skin, it should be promptly removed from the affected area using clean paper towels or cloth, followed by thorough rinsing with ample water.

3. Knowledge points

Knoevenagel condensation reaction, Michael addition reaction, the main sources of impurities in nitrendipine.

Ⅲ Experimental Equipments and Raw Materials

1. Experimental equipment

The condensation reaction apparatus is composed of a magnetic stirrer, an ice-water bath, a three-neck round-bottom flask, a thermometer, and a constant pressure funnel.

The addition reaction apparatus is composed of a magnetic stirrer, a three-neck round-bottom flask, and a thermometer.

The condensation reaction apparatus and the addition reaction apparatus

2. Raw materials

Synthetic product	Raw materials			
	Name	Quantity	Quality	Use
Ethyl 3-nitrobenzylideneacetoacetate	Ethyl acetoacetate	9. 8 g (0. 075 mol)	CP	Reactant
	Acetic anhydride	5. 1 g (0. 05 mol)	CP	Acylatant
	Concentrated sulfuric acid	0. 7 mL	CP	Catalyst
	3-Nitrobenzaldehyde	7. 7 g (0. 05 mol)	CP	Reactant
	Ethanol	10 mL	CP	Solvent
Nitrendipine	Ethyl 3-nitrobenzylideneacetoacetate	5. 3 g (0. 02 mol)	CP	Reactant
	Methyl 3-aminocrotonate	2. 8 g (0. 024 mol)	CP	Reactant
	Concentrated hydrochloric acid	0. 4 mL	CP	Catalyst
	Ethanol	18 mL	CP	Solvent

Ⅳ Procedure

1. Preparation of ethyl 3-nitrobenzylideneacetoacetate

(1) Add 9.8 g of ethyl acetoacetate and 5.1 g (4.8 mL) of acetic anhydride to a 100 mL three-necked flask. Cool to 0 ℃ in an ice-water bath, slowly add 1.2 g (0.7 mL) concentrated sulfuric acid dropwise with stirring for 10 min. Subsequently, add 7.7 g 3-nitrobenzaldehyde in 5 portions (ensuring that the temperature remains below 5 ℃).

(2) After adding, spontaneously raise the temperature to room temperature. The reaction solution becomes transparent and gradually becomes viscous and turbid. Keep it warm and stir for 1 h.

(3) Add 10 mL of 95% ethanol, stir and cool in an ice-water bath to 0~5 ℃, filter, and wash the solid twice with cold 95% ethanol (about 3 mL), then wash with cold water until pH=6.

(4) Let it dry in the air to obtain a white solid, weigh it, and calculate the yield.

2. Preparation of nitrendipine

(1) Add 5.3 g of ethyl 3-nitrobenzylidene acetoacetate, 2.8 g of methyl β-aminocrotonate, and 18 mL of anhydrous ethanol to a 100 mL three-necked flask in sequence. Install a reflux condenser and heat to reflux for 1 h.

(2) Add 0.4 mL of concentrated hydrochloric acid, continue to reflux for 0.5 h, cool slightly, add 10 mL of water dropwise, and cool in an ice-water bath until the solid precipitates completely.

(3) Filter and wash the filter cake 3~5 times with ice-cold 50% ethanol.

(4) Vacuum dry to obtain light yellow crystals, weigh it, measure the melting point, and calculate the yield.

(5) Send the final product to the place where the teachers designated.

Ⅴ Experimental Results

1. Yield

(1) Calculate the theoretical production of nitrendipine

$$\text{3-Nitrobenzaldehyde} \text{————} \text{Nitrendipine}$$
$$M_w = 151.12 \text{ g/mol} \text{————} M_w = 360.36 \text{ g/mol}$$
$$0.05 \text{ mol} \text{————} 0.05 \text{ mol}$$

Theoretical production $= 0.05 \text{ mol} \times 360.36 \text{ g/mol} = 18.02 \text{ g}$

(2) Calculate the percent yield of nitrendipine

$$\text{Yield} = \frac{\text{Practical production}}{\text{Theoretical production}} \times 100\% = \frac{(\quad)}{18.02 \text{ g}} \times 100\% = (\quad)\%$$

2. Appearance and melting point of product

A. Appearance: _____ ;

B. m. p. :

Theoretical value: 169~171 ℃;

Practical value: _____.

3. Analysis of experimental results

_____

_____

_____

_____

_____

_____

_____.

VI Notes

1. The presence of water impedes the advancement of reactions, necessitating the use of thoroughly dried instruments.

2. The speed of adding 3-nitrobenzaldehyde can be appropriately increased if the reaction temperature is controlled below 5 ℃.

3. When washing 3-nitrobenzyl acetoacetate, it is crucial to use approximately 3 mL of 95% ethanol per wash cycle. Excessive amounts can lead to partial dissolution of the product and adversely affect the overall yield, while insufficient quantities may impact the coloration of the final product.

4. The 50% ethanol should be pre-cooled to approximately −15 ℃ in order to prevent the dissolution of certain products.

VII Determination of Product Content

Titration method. Take about 0.13 g of this product, weigh it accurately, add 20 mL of acetic acid and 10 mL of dilute sulfuric acid, dissolve at a low temperature, and let cool. Add $2 \sim 3$ drops of orthophenanthroline indicator solution, slowly titrate with cerium sulfate titrant (0.1 mol/L) until the red color disappears, and calibrate the titration results with the blank test solution. Each 1 mL of cerium sulfate titrant (0.1 mol/L) is equivalent to 18.02 mg of nitrendipine. (Chinese Pharmacopoeia 2020 Edition)

VIII Discussion Questions

1. What is the primary function of acetic anhydride in the reaction? Can it be replaced by other reagents?

2. What role does concentrated sulfuric acid play in the reaction? Can it be replaced by other acids?

3. Please briefly describe the principle of the Michael addition reaction.

(By Yingchao Duan)

实验十一

尼群地平的合成

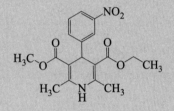

背景知识

尼群地平为第二代 1,4-二氢吡啶类钙通道阻滞药，1985 年于德国首次上市，主要用于治疗高血压、充血性心力衰竭和伴有心绞痛的高血压（图 11-1）。尼群地平能选择性作用于血管平滑肌的 L 亚型钙通道，抑制血管平滑肌和心肌的跨膜钙离子内流，其对血管的亲和力比对心肌大，对冠状动脉的选择作用更强；能降低心肌耗氧量，对缺血心肌有保护作用；可降低总外周阻力，使血压下降。

图 11-1 尼群地平的化学结构

尼群地平的作用机制

I 目的与要求

1. 掌握尼群地平的合成操作。
2. 熟悉 Knoevenagel 缩合反应和迈克尔加成的反应原理。
3. 了解尼群地平中杂质的主要来源。

II 实验原理

1. 主要反应物及产物的物理常数

名称	结构式 CAS 号	分子式 分子量	熔点或 沸点/℃	溶解性
3-硝基苯甲醛	99-61-6	$C_7H_5NO_3$ 151.12	m. p. 56~59	20 ℃水中溶解度为 1.6 mg/mL，易溶于常用有机溶剂
乙酰乙酸乙酯	141-97-9	$C_6H_{10}O_3$ 130.14	b. p. 180.8	20 ℃水中溶解度为 2.86 g/100 mL，易溶于常用有机溶剂

名称	结构式 CAS 号	分子式 分子量	熔点或沸点/℃	溶解性
乙酸酐	H₃C—O—CH₃ 108-24-7	$C_4H_6O_3$ 102.09	b. p. 140	缓慢溶于水形成乙酸,易溶于氯仿和乙醚
β-氨基巴豆酸甲酯	14205-39-1	$C_5H_9NO_2$ 115.13	m. p. 81~83	易溶于常用有机溶剂
3-硝基亚苄基乙酰乙酸乙酯	39562-16-8	$C_{13}H_{13}NO_5$ 263.25	m. p. 162~164	不溶于水,易溶于丙酮、二氯甲烷、氯仿等,微溶于甲醇,乙醇
尼群地平	39562-70-4	$C_{18}H_{20}N_2O_6$ 360.36	m. p. 169~171	不溶于水,易溶于丙酮、二氯甲烷、氯仿等,微溶于甲醇,乙醇

2. 合成路线

3-硝基苯甲醛 + 乙酰乙酸乙酯 $\xrightarrow[\text{H}_2\text{SO}_4]{(CH_3CO)_2O}$ 3-硝基亚苄基乙酰乙酸乙酯

$\xrightarrow{\text{HCl, } C_2H_5OH}$ 尼群地平

尼群地平的合成以 3-硝基苯甲醛和乙酰乙酸乙酯为原料,在乙酸酐和浓硫酸存在下,通过缩合反应获得中间体,然后,经迈克尔加成和环合反应获得目标化合物。环合反应过程中,在 70 ℃和酸性条件下,二氢吡啶环易发生氧化反应生成吡啶类副产物。此外,在 70 ℃和酸性条件下,还易发生酯交换反应,生成少量双甲酯副产物和双乙酯副产物。

吡啶类副产物   双甲酯副产物   双乙酯副产物

安全提示：乙酸酐、浓盐酸可灼伤皮肤，并有刺激性气味，应在通风橱中使用。乙酸酐、浓盐酸一旦接触皮肤，要立即用大量水冲洗。浓硫酸接触皮肤后，用干净的纸巾或者毛巾将局部皮肤上的浓硫酸迅速清除掉，然后再用大量的清水局部冲洗。

3. 知识点

Knoevenagel 缩合反应，迈克尔加成，尼群地平中杂质的主要来源。

环合反应
装置和加成
反应装置

Ⅲ 实验装置和原料

1. 实验装置

环合反应装置由磁力搅拌器、冰水浴、三口烧瓶、温度计和恒压滴液漏斗组成。加成反应装置由磁力搅拌器、三口烧瓶和温度计组成。

2. 原料

合成产物	原料			
	名称	用量	试剂级别	用途
3-硝基亚苄基乙酰乙酸乙酯	乙酰乙酸乙酯	9.8 g(0.075 mol)	化学纯	反应物
	乙酸酐	5.1 g(0.05 mol)	化学纯	酰化试剂
	浓硫酸	0.7 mL	化学纯	催化剂
	3-硝基苯甲醛	7.7 g(0.05 mol)	化学纯	反应物
	乙醇	10 mL	化学纯	溶剂
尼群地平	3-硝基亚苄基乙酰乙酸乙酯	5.3 g(0.02 mol)	化学纯	反应物
	β-氨基巴豆酸甲酯	2.8 g(0.024 mol)	化学纯	反应物
	浓盐酸	0.4 mL	化学纯	催化剂
	乙醇	18 mL	化学纯	溶剂

Ⅳ 实验操作

1. 3-硝基亚苄基乙酰乙酸乙酯的制备

（1）在装有磁力搅拌器、温度计和恒压滴液漏斗的 100 mL 三口烧瓶中，依次加入 9.8 g 乙酰乙酸乙酯和 5.1 g(4.8 mL) 乙酸酐，用冰水浴冷却至 0℃，搅拌下缓慢滴加 1.2 g(0.7 mL) 浓硫酸，10 min 后，分 5 批加入（其间保持温度不超过 5℃）7.7 g 3-硝基苯甲醛。

（2）加毕，自然升温至室温，反应液透明并逐渐变得黏稠、浑浊，保温搅拌 1 h。

（3）加入 10 mL 95％乙醇，搅拌下冰水浴冷却至 0～5℃，抽滤，所得固体用冷 95％乙醇（约 3 mL）洗涤 2 次，再用冷水洗涤至 pH 为 6。

（4）自然晾干，得类白色固体，称重，计算收率。

2. 尼群地平的制备

（1）100 mL 三口烧瓶中依次加入 5.3 g 3-硝基亚苄基乙酰乙酸乙酯、2.8 g β-氨基巴豆酸甲酯和 18 mL 无水乙醇，安装回流冷凝装置，加热回流 1 h。

（2）加入 0.4 mL 浓盐酸，继续回流 0.5 h，稍冷，滴加 10 mL 水，冰水浴冷却至固体析出完全。

（3）抽滤，滤饼用冰冷的 50％乙醇洗涤 3～5 次。

（4）真空干燥，得淡黄色晶体，称重，测熔点，计算收率。

（5）将产物送到指导教师指定的产品回收处。

V 实验结果

1. 收率

（1）计算尼群地平的理论产量。

$$3\text{-硝基苯甲醛} \longrightarrow \text{尼群地平}$$
$$M_w = 151.12 \text{ g/mol} \longrightarrow M_w = 360.36 \text{ g/mol}$$
$$0.05 \text{ mol} \longrightarrow 0.05 \text{ mol}$$
$$\text{理论产量} = 0.05 \text{ mol} \times 360.36 \text{ g/mol} = 18.02 \text{ g}$$

（2）计算尼群地平的收率

$$\text{收率} = \frac{\text{产品实际产量}}{\text{产品理论产量}} \times 100\% = \frac{(\quad\quad)}{18.02 \text{ g}} \times 100\% = (\quad\quad)\%$$

2. 产品外观与熔点

A. 外观：_____；

B. 熔点：

理论值：169～171 ℃；

实测值：_____。

3. 实验结果分析

_____

_____

_____

_____

_____

_____

_____。

VI 注意事项

1. 两步反应中，水都会影响反应的进行，因此所有仪器应干燥。

2. 加入 3-硝基苯甲醛时，只要反应温度能控制在 5 ℃以下，可以适当加快加入速度。

3. 洗涤 3-硝基亚苄基乙酰乙酸乙酯时，冷 95％乙醇每次用量大约 3 mL，用量太多会溶解部分产品，影响收率，用量太少会影响产品的色泽。

4.50%乙醇最好预先冷却至−15 ℃左右，否则会溶解部分产品。

Ⅶ 产物的含量测定

滴定法：取本品约 0.13 g，精密称定，加冰醋酸 20 mL 及稀硫酸 10 mL，微温使溶解，放冷；加邻二氮菲指示液 2～3 滴，用硫酸铈滴定液（0.1 mol/L）缓缓滴定至红色消失，并将滴定的结果用空白试液校正。每 1 mL 的硫酸铈滴定液（0.1 mol/L）相当于 18.02 mg 的尼群地平。（《中华人民共和国药典（2020年版）》）

Ⅷ 思考题

1. 乙酸酐在反应中所起的主要作用是什么？能否用其他试剂代替？
2. 浓硫酸在反应中起什么作用？能否用其他酸代替？
3. 简述迈克尔加成反应的原理。

（段迎超）

The mechanism
of action of
Ciprofloxacin

Experiment 12

Synthesis of Ciprofloxacin Monohydrochloride Monohydrate

Background

Ciprofloxacin is a third-generation quinolone antibiotic. It is developed and marketed by Bayer Pharmaceuticals in Germany and its commercial name is "Ciprobay". The chemical structure of ciprofloxacin is shown in Fig. 12-1.

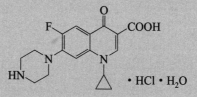

Fig. 12-1　Structure of Ciprofloxacin

Ⅰ　Purposes and Requirements

1. To master the principles and operation requirements of cyclization，hydrolysis and *N*-alkylation reaction.

2. To strengthen the anhydrous reaction operation.

3. To understand the interaction between ciprofloxacin hydrochloride and target.

Ⅱ　Principle of the Reaction

1. Physical data of the main reactants and product

Name	Structure CAS No.	Formula M. Wt	b. p. or m. p. /℃	Solubility
Methyl 3-（cyclopropylamino)-2-（2,4-dichloro-5-fluorobenzoyl)acrylate(compound **2**)	105392-26-5	$C_{14}H_{12}Cl_2FNO_3$ 332. 15	m. p. 156～158	—

Name	Structure CAS No.	Formula M. Wt	b. p. or m. p. /℃	Solubility
3-Quinolinecarboxylic acid, 7-chloro-1-cyclopropyl-6-fluoro-1,4-dihydro-4-oxo-, Methyl ester(compound **3**)	104599-90-8	$C_{14}H_{11}ClFNO_3$ 295.69	m. p. 256	—
7-Chloro-1-cyclopropyl-6-fluoro-1,4-dihydro-4-oxoquinoline-3-carboxylic acid(compound **4**)	86393-33-1	$C_{13}H_9Cl_2FNO_3$ 281.67	m. p. 245~246	—
Ciprofloxacin(compound **5**)	85721-33-1	$C_{17}H_{18}FN_3O_3$ 331.34	m. p. 255~257	—
Ciprofloxacin monohydrochloride monohydrate(compound **1**)	86393-32-0	$C_{17}H_{18}FN_3O_3 \cdot$ $HCl \cdot H_2O$ 385.82	m. p. 318~320	Well soluble in water
Potassium carbonate	K_2CO_3 584-08-7	K_2CO_3 138.21	m. p. 891	Well soluble in water
DMF	68-12-2	C_3H_7NO 73.09	b. p. 153	Soluble in water and most organic solvents
Piperazine	110-85-0	$C_4H_{10}N_2$ 86.14	m. p. 107~111	Soluble in water, methanol, and ethanol; slightly soluble in benzene, ether
3-Methyl-1-butanol	123-51-3	$C_5H_{12}O$ 88.15	b. p. 132.5	Slightly soluble in water; soluble in ethanol, ether, benzene, chloroform, and petroleum ether; well soluble in acetone

Experiment 12　Synthesis of Ciprofloxacin Monohydrochloride Monohydrate ┃ 115

2. Synthetic route

Methyl 3-(cyclopropylamino)-
2-(2,4-dichloro-5-
fluorobenzoyl)acrylate(**2**)

$\xrightarrow[\text{DMF}]{\text{K}_2\text{CO}_3}$

3-Quinolinecarboxylic acid,
7-chloro-1-cyclopropyl-6-
fluoro-1,4-dihydro-4-oxo-,
Methyl ester(**3**)

$\xrightarrow[\text{(2) H}^+]{\text{(1) OH}^-}$

7-Chloro-1-cyclopropyl-6-
fluoro-1,4-dihydro-4-
oxoquinoline-3-carboxylic acid(**4**)

(1) HN⌒NH
(2) isoamyl alcohol OH

Ciprofloxacin(**5**)

$\xrightarrow[\text{CH}_3\text{CH}_2\text{OH}]{\text{HCl, H}_2\text{O}}$

• HCl • H$_2$O

Ciprofloxacin monohydrochloride
monohydrate(**1**)

The synthesis of ciprofloxacin hydrochloride involves using cyclopropylamine compound as raw materials, followed by cyclization, hydrolysis, piperazination, and salt formation reactions to obtain the target compound.

Safety Tips: The cyclization reaction step requires heating DMF to 140 ℃. Due to the high temperature and alkaline conditions, DMF is prone to decompose and produce dimethylamine and carbon monoxide gas. It is important to note that the reaction apparatus should be open.

3. Knowledge points

Cyclization reaction, hydrolysis reaction, *N*-alkylation reaction, anhydrous reaction operation.

Ⅲ Experimental Equipments and Raw Materials

1. Experimental equipments

The cyclization reaction apparatus is composed of a magnetic stirrer, a three-neck round-bottom flask, a spherical condenser tube, a thermometer, and a drying tube.

The hydrolysis reaction apparatus is composed of a magnetic stirrer, a three-

The cyclization
reaction
apparatus
and the
hydrolysis
reaction
apparatus

neck round-bottom flask, a spherical condenser tube, and a thermometer.

2. Raw materials

Synthetic product	Raw materials			
	Name	Quantity	Quality	Use
3-Quinolinecarboxylic acid, 7-chloro-1-cyclopropyl-6-fluoro-1,4-dihydro-4-oxo-, Methyl ester(compound **3**)	Methyl 3-(cyclopropylamino)-2-(2,4-dichloro-5-fluorobenzoyl) acrylate	5 g	Product prepared	Reactant
	Potassium carbonate anhydrous	3.17 g (0.023 mol)	CP	Reactant
	DMF	39 mL	CP	Solvent
	Water	50 mL	—	Solid precipitation
7-Chloro-1-cyclopropyl-6-fluoro-1,4-dihydro-4-oxoquinoline-3-carboxylic acid (compound **4**)	3-Quinolinecarboxylic acid, 7-chloro-1-cyclopropyl-6-fluoro-1,4-dihydro-4-oxo-, Methyl ester	Proper amount	Product prepared	Reactant
	Sodium hydroxide	1.8 g (0.045 mol)	CP	Reactant
	Hydrochloric acid	Proper amount	CP	Adjusting pH
	Distilled water	34 mL	—	Solvent
Ciprofloxacin monohydrochloride monohydrate(compound **1**)	7-Chloro-1-cyclopropyl-6-fluoro-1,4-dihydro-4-oxoquinoline-3-carboxylic acid	4 g (0.014 mol)	Product prepared	Reactant
	Piperazine anhydrous	4.8 g (0.056 mol)	CP	Reactant
	isoamyl ethanol	30 mL	CP	Solvent
	95% Ethanol	50 mL	CP	Solvent
	Concentrated hydrochloric acid	Proper amount	CP	Reactant
	Distilled water	Proper amount	—	Solvent
	Activated carbon	0.5 g	CP	Discolouring agent

Ⅳ Operations

1. Preparation of methyl 7-chloro-1-cyclopropyl-6-fluoro-4-oxo-1,4-dihydro-quinoline-3-carboxylate(compound 3)

(1) Equip the cyclization reaction apparatus.

(2) Add 5 g methyl 3-(cyclopropylamino)-2-(2,4-dichloro-5-fluorobenzoyl) acrylate, 3.17 g anhydrous potassium carbonate and 39 mL DMF into a 100 mL three neck round bottom flask.

(3) Heat up the mixture to 140 ℃ and keep for 1.5 h.

(4) The mixture should be cooled to 50 ℃. Add 50 mL of water to the above reaction mixture, precipitate solid particles, filter and wash with water to obtain crude product. The crude product can be directly used in the next reaction.

2. Preparation of 7-chloro-1-cyclopropyl-6-fluoro-1,4-dihydro-4-oxoquinoline-3-carboxylic acid(compound 4)

(1) Equip the hydrolysis reaction apparatus.

Experimental operation of cyclization reaction (video)

Experimental procedure of cyclization reaction

Experimental
operation of
hydrolysis
reaction（video）

Experimental
procedure of
hydrolysis
reaction

Experimental
operation of
N-alkylation
reaction（video）

Experimental
procedure of
N-alkylation
reaction

（2）A solution composed of the above cyclic product，1. 8 g sodium hydroxide and 34 mL distilled water are added to a 250 mL three-neck round-bottom flask and heat to 95～100 ℃ and maintain at this temperature for 1. 5 h.

（3）Then，cool the mixture to 50 ℃. Adjust the pH to 1 with concentrated hydrochloric acid，raise the reaction temperature to 80 ℃，maintain for 30 min，and cool to room temperature.

（4）Filter and wash the filtrate with water to neutralize the acid. Dry the product under an infrared lamp. Weigh the product and calculate the yield. Measure the melting point. If the melting point does not match，recrystallization is needed.

（5）The recrystallization conditions are as follows：dissolve the crude product in 5 times DMF with heating. Add activated carbon and reheat. Filter while it is hot to remove activated carbon and crystallize by cooling. Filter it and wash the filtrate with DMF. Dry the product under an infrared lamp.

3. Preparation of ciprofloxacin monohydrochloride monohydrate （compound 1）

（1）Equip the cyclization reaction apparatus.

（2）Add 4 g of the product obtained above，4. 8 g anhydrous piperazine and 30 mL isoamyl ethanol into the 100 mL three-neck round-bottom flask.

（3）Heat the mixture to reflux and maintain for 6 h. Cool the mixture to 10 ℃，precipitate the solid particles，filter and wash with water.

（4）Dissolve the solid product obtained in 20 mL of 10％ hydrochloric acid，reflux with activated carbon for 30 minutes and filter while it is hot.

（5）Cool the filtrate to 65 ℃，add 95％ ethanol，reflux to transparent，cool it again to 10～15 ℃，precipitate and filter.

（6）Dry the product under an infrared lamp and weigh it up. Calculate the yield and measure the melting point.

（7）Send the final product to the place where the teachers designated.

Ⅴ Experimental Results

1. Yield

（1）Calculate the theoretical production of ciprofloxacin monohydrochloride monohydrate

Cyclopropylamine ———— Ciprofloxacin monohydrochloride monohydrate

M_w＝332. 15 g/mol ————M_w＝385. 82 g/mol

0. 015 mol ————0. 015 mol

Theoretical production＝0. 015 mol×385. 82 g/mol＝5. 79 g

（2）Calculate the percent yield of ciprofloxacin monohydrochloride monohydrate

$$\text{Yield}=\frac{\text{Practical production}}{\text{Theoretical production}}\times100\%=\frac{(\qquad)}{5.79\text{ g}}\times100\%=(\qquad)\%$$

2. Appearance and melting point of product

A. Appearance：＿＿＿＿＿＿＿＿＿＿＿＿＿＿＿＿＿＿＿＿＿＿；

B. m. p. ：

Theoretical value: 318~320 ℃;

Practical value: _____ .

3. Analysis of experimental results

_____
_____
_____
_____
_____
_____
_____ .

Ⅵ Notes

1. The control of reaction temperature in each step is an important factor.

2. The whole reaction takes place in a sequence whereby the product of the one step will be used in the next step. So, the amount of reagent used should be calculated proportionally.

Ⅶ Determination of Product Content

Chromatographic conditions: using octadecylsilane bonded silica gel as the filler. Using 0.025 mol/L phosphoric acid solution acetonitrile (87 : 13) (adjusted to pH 3.0 ± 0.1 with triethylamine) as the mobile phase. The flow rate is 1.5 mL per minute. The detection wavelength is 278 nm. The injection volume is 20 μL.

Measurement method: High-performance liquid chromatography method. Accurately weigh the test sample and reference solution, inject them separately into the liquid chromatograph, and record the chromatogram. Calculate the content of ciprofloxacin in the test sample based on peak area using the external standard method. (《Chinese Pharmacopoeia》 2020 Edition)

Ⅷ Discussion Questions

1. In terms of structure, what substances can be used instead of isoamyl ethanol?

2. In terms of structure, what substances are the by-product of the piperazine reaction of the 6-fluoro in the condensation reaction of piperazine?

(By Yichao Zheng)

实验十二

盐酸环丙沙星的合成

背景知识

环丙沙星（Ciprofloxacin），也称作环丙氟哌酸，为第三代喹诺酮类抗菌药物，由德国拜耳医药开发上市，商品名为"西普乐"，其化学结构见图 12-1。

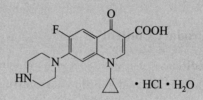

图 12-1 环丙沙星化学结构

环丙沙星的作用机制

I 目的与要求

1. 掌握环合反应、水解反应、*N*-烷基化反应的原理和操作要求。
2. 进一步巩固无水反应操作。
3. 了解盐酸环丙沙星与靶标的作用方式。

II 实验原理

1. 主要反应物和产物的物理常数

名称	结构式 CAS 号	分子式 分子量	沸点或 熔点/℃	溶解度
2-(2,4-二氯-5-氟苯甲酰)-3-环丙胺基丙烯酸甲酯（化合物 **2**）	105392-26-5	$C_{14}H_{12}Cl_2FNO_3$ 332.15	m. p. 156～158	—
1-环丙基-7-氯-6-氟-1,4-二氢-4-氧代喹啉-3-羧酸甲酯（化合物 **3**）	104599-90-8	$C_{14}H_{11}ClFNO_3$ 295.69	m. p. 256	—

名称	结构式 CAS 号	分子式 分子量	沸点或 熔点/℃	溶解度
1-环丙基-7-氯-6-氟- 1,4-二氢-4-氧代喹啉- 3-羧酸(化合物 4)	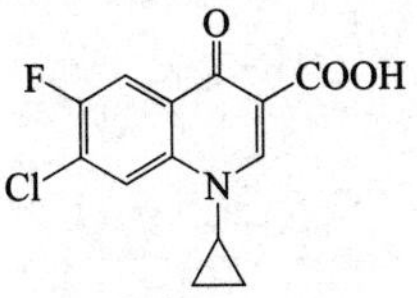 86393-33-1	$C_{13}H_9Cl_2FNO_3$ 281.67	m. p. 245～246	—
环丙沙星 (化合物 5)	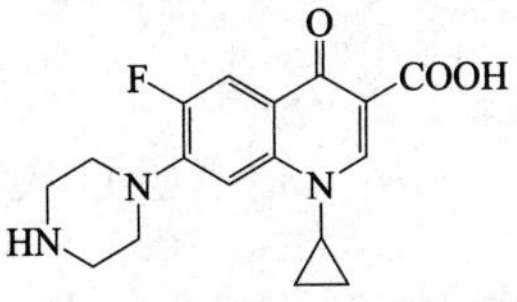 85721-33-1	$C_{17}H_{18}FN_3O_3$ 331.34	m. p. 255～257	—
盐酸环丙沙星 (化合物 1)	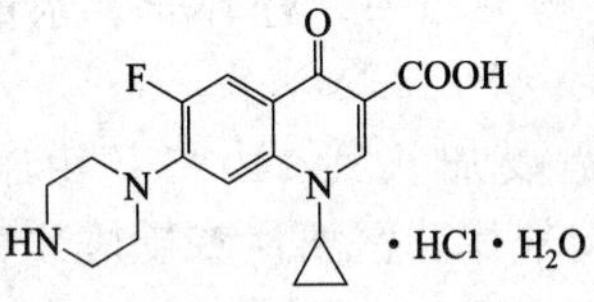 86393-32-0	$C_{17}H_{18}FN_3O_3 \cdot$ $HCl \cdot H_2O$ 385.82	m. p. 318～320	易溶于水
碳酸钾	K_2CO_3 584-08-7	K_2CO_3 138.21	m. p. 891	易溶于水
DMF	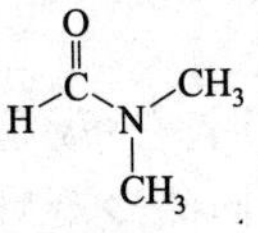 68-12-2	C_3H_7NO 73.09	b. p. 153	和水及大部分有机溶剂互溶
无水哌嗪	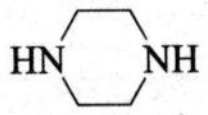 110-85-0	$C_4H_{10}N_2$ 86.14	m. p. 107～111	溶于水、甲醇、乙醇,微溶于苯、乙醚
异戊醇	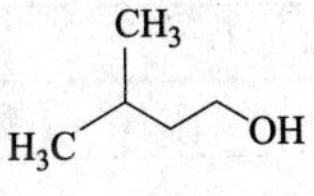 123-51-3	$C_5H_{12}O$ 88.15	b. p. 132.5	微溶于水,可混溶于乙醇、乙醚、苯、氯仿、石油醚,易溶于丙酮

2. 合成路线

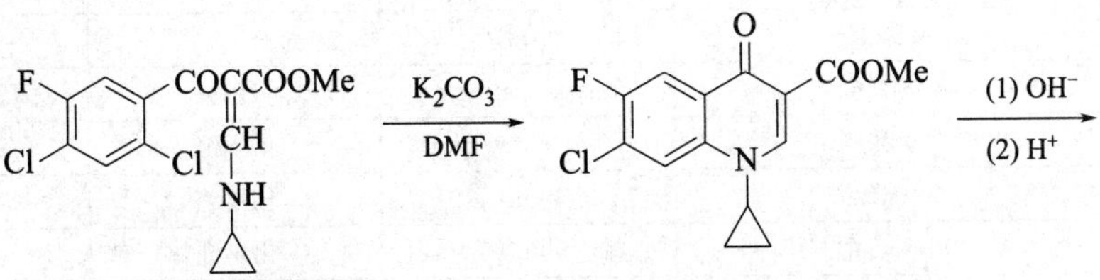

2-(2,4-二氯-5-氟苯甲酰)-
3-环丙胺基丙烯酸甲酯
(2)

$\xrightarrow[\text{DMF}]{K_2CO_3}$

1-环丙基-7-氯-6-氟-1,4-
二氢-4-氧代喹啉-3-羧酸甲酯
(3)

$\xrightarrow{\begin{array}{l}(1)\ OH^-\\(2)\ H^+\end{array}}$

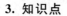

1-环丙基-7-氯-6-氟-1,4-
二氢-4-氧代喹啉-3-羧酸
（**4**）

环丙沙星
（**5**）

盐酸环丙沙星一水合物（**1**）

盐酸环丙沙星的合成，以环丙胺化物为原料，经环合、水解和哌嗪化和成盐反应得到目标物。

安全提示：环合反应步骤，DMF 需要加热到 140 ℃，由于高温和碱性条件下，DMF 易分解生产二甲胺和一氧化碳气体，需要注意反应装置不能密闭。

3. 知识点

环合反应，水解反应，*N*-烷基化反应，无水反应操作。

Ⅲ 实验装置和原料

环合反应
装置和水解
反应装置

1. 实验装置

环合反应装置由磁力搅拌器、三口烧瓶、回流冷凝管、温度计和干燥管组成。水解反应装置由磁力搅拌器、三口烧瓶、回流冷凝管和温度计组成。

2. 原料

合成产物	原料			
	名称	用量	试剂级别	用途
1-环丙基-7-氯-6-氟-1,4-二氢-4-氧代喹啉-3-羧酸甲酯（化合物 **3**）	环丙胺化物	5 g	自制	反应物
	无水碳酸钾	3.17 g（0.023 mol）	化学纯	反应物
	DMF	39 mL	化学纯	溶剂
	水	50 mL	—	析出固体
1-环丙基-7-氯-6-氟-1,4-二氢-4-氧代喹啉-3-羧酸（化合物 **4**）	环化物	适量	自制	反应物
	氢氧化钠	1.8 g（0.045 mol）	化学纯	反应物
	盐酸	适量	化学纯	调节 pH 值
	蒸馏水	34 mL	—	溶剂
盐酸环丙沙星（化合物 **1**）	环丙羧酸	4 g（0.014 mol）	自制	反应物
	无水哌嗪	4.8 g（0.056 mol）	化学纯	反应物
	异戊醇	30 mL	化学纯	溶剂
	95 % 乙醇	50 mL	化学纯	溶剂
	浓盐酸	适量	化学纯	反应物
	蒸馏水	适量	—	溶剂
	活性炭	0.5 g	化学纯	脱色剂

Ⅳ 实验操作

1. 1-环丙基-7-氯-6-氟-1，4-二氢-4-氧代喹啉-3-羧酸甲酯（化合物3）合成

（1）搭建环合反应装置。

（2）于 100 mL 三口烧瓶中，加入 5 g 化合物 **2**、3.17 g 无水碳酸钾和 39 mL DMF。

（3）升温至 140 ℃反应 1.5 h。

（4）降温至 50 ℃，在以上体系中，加入 50 mL 水，析出固体，抽滤，水洗，得粗品，粗品直接用于下一步反应。

环合反应的
实验操作
（视频）

2. 1-环丙基-7-氯-6-氟-1，4-二氢-4-氧代喹啉-3-羧酸（化合物4）合成

（1）搭建水解反应装置。

（2）在 250 mL 三口烧瓶中，加入化合物 **3**、1.8 g 氢氧化钠和 34 mL 蒸馏水配成的溶液，升温至 95～100 ℃反应 1.5 h。

（3）冷却至 50 ℃。然后，用浓盐酸调 pH＝1，升温至 80 ℃反应 0.5 h，冷却至室温。

（4）过滤，水洗至中性，烘干，测熔点（234～237 ℃）。若熔点不符，则需重结晶，计算收率。

（5）重结晶的条件为：取粗品，用 5 倍量的 DMF，加热溶解，加入活性炭，再次加热，过滤，除去活性炭，冷却，结晶，抽滤，洗涤，烘干得产品。

水解反应的
实验操作
（视频）

3. 盐酸环丙沙星（化合物1）合成

（1）搭建环合反应装置。

（2）在 100 mL 三口烧瓶中，加入 4 g 化合物 **4**、4.8 g 无水哌嗪和 30 mL 异戊醇。

（3）升温至回流反应 6 h。冷却至 10 ℃，析出固体，抽滤，水洗。

（4）将所获得的固体溶于 10 ％盐酸 20 mL 中，加活性炭回流 0.5 h，热过滤。

（5）滤液冷却至 65 ℃，加入 95 ％乙醇，继续回流至透明，冷却至 10～15 ℃，析出固体，抽滤。

（6）烘干纯品，称重，计算收率，测熔点。

（7）将产物送到指导教师指定的产品回收处。

N-烷基化
反应的实验
操作（视频）

Ⅴ 实验结果

1. 收率

（1）计算盐酸环丙沙星的理论产量

$$环丙胺化物 \text{————} 盐酸环丙沙星$$

$$M_w＝332.15 \text{ g/mol} \text{————} M_w＝385.82 \text{ g/mol}$$

$$0.015 \text{ mol} \text{————} 0.015 \text{ mol}$$

$$理论产量＝0.015 \text{ mol} \times 385.82 \text{ g/mol}＝5.79 \text{ g}$$

（2）计算盐酸环丙沙星的收率

$$收率＝\frac{产品实际产量}{产品理论产量} \times 100 ＝\frac{(\quad)}{5.79 \text{ g}} \times 100 ＝(\quad)$$

2. 产品外观与熔点

A. 外观：＿＿＿＿＿＿＿＿＿＿；

B. 熔点：

    理论值：318～320℃

    实测值：_____。

3. 实验结果分析

_____

_____

_____

_____

_____

_____

_____

_____。

Ⅵ 注意事项

1. 各步骤反应温度控制是重要的因素。

2. 整个反应是接着上一步反应进行的，所用试剂的量需要按照比例计算后使用。

Ⅶ 产物的含量测定

色谱条件： 用十八烷基硅烷键合硅胶为填充剂；以 0.025 mol/L 磷酸溶液-乙腈（87：13）（用三乙胺调节 pH 值至 3.0±0.1）为流动相；流速为每分钟 1.5 mL；检测波长为 278 nm；进样体积 20 μL。

测定法： 采用高效液相色谱法。精密量取供试品与对照品溶液，分别注入液相色谱仪，记录色谱图。按外标法以峰面积计算供试品中环丙沙星的含量。（《中华人民共和国药典（2020 年版)》）

Ⅷ 思考题

1. 用结构式表示，所用异戊醇还可以用什么代替？

2. 哌嗪化反应时，6-氟发生哌嗪化副产物的结构式是什么？

（郑一超）

Experiment 13

Synthesis of Phenytoin Sodium

Background

Phenytoin sodium, also known as dilantin, is a preferred antiepileptic drug for tonic-clonic seizures, and can also be used as an antiarrhythmic drug. The chemical structure of phenytoin sodium is shown in Fig. 13-1.

The mechanism of action of Phenytoin sodium

Fig. 13-1　Structure of Phenytoin Sodium

I　Purposes and Requirements

1. To master the principle and operation requirements of the benzoin condensation reaction, oxidation reaction and rearrangement reaction.

2. To understand the interaction between phenytoin sodium and target.

II　Principle of the Reaction

1. Physical data of the main reactants and product

Name	Structure CAS No.	Formula M. Wt	b. p. or m. p. /℃	Solubility
Benzaldehyde	100-52-7	C_7H_6O 106. 12	b. p. 179	Water: <0. 01 g/100 mL
Benzoin	119-53-9	$C_{14}H_{12}O_2$ 212. 24	m. p. 134~138	Insoluble in water, slightly soluble in ethers, soluble in ethanols

Name	Structure CAS No.	Formula M. Wt	b. p. or m. p. /℃	Solubility
1-Phenyl-1,2-propanedione	579-07-7	$C_9H_8O_2$ 210.23	m. p. 95~96	Soluble in ethanol, ether, acetone, benzene, and chloroform; insoluble in water
Phenytoin	57-41-0	$C_{15}H_{12}N_2O_2$ 252.27	m. p. 293~295	In water: <0.01 g/100 mL; soluble in DMSO
Phenytoin sodium	630-93-3	$C_{15}H_{11}NaO_2$ 274.25	m. p. 292~299	Well soluble in water; soluble in ethanol; insoluble in chloroform
Thiamine hydrochloride (Vitamin B$_1$)	67-03-8	$C_{12}H_{16}N_4OS \cdot$ HCl 337.27	m. p. 245~250	Well soluble in water; slightly soluble in ethanol; insoluble in ether, benzene, chloroform and acetone
Ferric chloride hexahydrate	$FeCl_3 \cdot 6H_2O$ 10025-77-1	$FeCl_3 \cdot 6H_2O$ 270.30	m. p. 37	Well soluble in water
Urea	NH_2CONH_2 57-13-6	CH_4N_2O 60.06	m. p. 132.7	Soluble in water, methanol, formal-dehyde, ethanol, solution ammonia, and ethanol; slightly soluble in ether, chloroform, benzene

2. Synthetic route

Benzaldehyde → (Vitamin B$_1$) → Benzoin → (FeCl$_3$ · 6H$_2$O) → 1-Phenyl-1,2-propanedione

(1) NH$_2$CONH$_2$, NaOH (2) HCl → 5,5-Diphenylhydantoin → NaOH → Phenytoin sodium

Benzoin is obtained from benzaldehyde by the benzoin condensation reaction which uses vitamin B$_1$ as a cofactor. Benzoin then undergoes oxidation to form 1,2-

diphenylethylene ketone. Phenytoin is then synthesized by condensation and rear rangement reactions from urea in alkaline conditions. Finally, sodium phenytoin is prepared by the salt formation reaction.

Safety Tips: Benzaldehyde can stimulate the mucosa of the eyes and respiratory tract.

3. Knowledge points

Benzoin condensation reaction, oxidation reaction, rearrangement reaction, reaction mechanism.

Ⅲ Experimental Equipment and Raw Materials

The reaction
apparatus

1. Experimental equipment

The reaction apparatus is composed of a magnetic stirrer, a three-neck round-bottom flask, a spherical condenser tube and a thermometer.

2. Raw materials

Synthetic product	Raw materials			
	Name	Quantity	Quality	Use
Benzoin	Benzaldehyde	10 mL (0. 098 mol)	CP	Reactant
	Thiamine hydrochloride (Vitamin B$_1$)	1. 75 g(0. 005 mol)	CP(60 %)	Catalytic agent
	95 % ethanol	15 mL	—	Solvent
	2 mol/L NaOH	5 mL	—	Catalytic agent
	Distilled water	Proper amount	—	Solvent
1-Phenyl-1,2-propanedione	Benzoin	2. 12 g (0. 010 mol)	Product prepared	Reactant
	Ferric chloride hexahydrate	9. 0 g (0. 033 mol)	CP	Oxidizing agent
	Glacial acetic acid	10 mL	CP	Solvent
	95 % Ethanol	Proper amount	CP	Solvent
	Distilled water	Proper amount	—	Solvent
	Ethyl ether	Proper amount	CP	Solvent
Phenytoin	1-Phenyl-1,2-propanedione	1 g	Product prepared	Reactant
	Urea	0. 57 g (0. 0095 mol)	CP	Reactant
	15 % NaOH	3. 1 mL	Product prepared	Catalytic agent
	95 % Ethanol	5 mL	CP	Solvent
	15 % Hydrochloric acid	proper amount	—	Neutralization reagent
	Distilled water	37 mL	—	Solvent
Phenytoin sodium	Phenytoin	1 g	Product prepared	Reactant
	15 % NaOH	5 mL	Product prepared	Reactant
	Activated carbon	Proper amount	CP	Discolouring agent
	Distilled water	5 mL	—	Solvent

IV Operations

1. Preparation of benzoin

(1) Equip the reaction apparatus.

(2) Add 1.75 g Vitamin B_1 and 4 mL distilled water into the 50 mL three-neck round-bottom flask, and dissolve by stirring. Add 15 mL 95% ethanol to this solution, and 5 mL sodium hydroxide solution (2 mol/L) dropwise. Stir the reaction solution at room temperature for 5 min. Next, add 10 mL benzaldehyde and stir evenly. Keep this reaction mixture at room temperature for 1 week.

(3) Finally, filter the above system, wash the filter cake with a small amount of ice water, dry and weigh it up. Calculate the the yield and measure the melting point.

2. Preparation of 1-phenyl-1,2-propanedione

(1) Equip the reaction apparatus.

(2) Add 2.12 g benzoin, 9.0 g ferric chloride hexahydrate and 5 mL water into the 100 mL three-neck round-bottom flask, and stir evenly. Add 10 mL glacial acetic acid, and heat the mixture to reflux and maintain for 1 h. Then, add 50 mL water and continue heating and refluxing for 5 min.

(3) Cool the mixture to room temperature, and let the solid precipitate and filter. The filter cake is crude 1,2-diphenylacetone.

(4) Recrystallize the crude product with 12 mL ethanol, and filter, wash with a small amount of cold ethanol-ether solution, dry and weigh. Calculate the yield and measure the melting point.

3. Preparation of phenytoin

(1) Equip the reaction apparatus.

(2) Add 1 g 1-phenyl-1,2- propanedione, 0.57 g urea, 3.1 mL 15% sodium hydroxide and 5 mL ethanol into a 100 mL three-neck round-bottom flask, heat the mixture to reflux for 2 h, and cool down to room temperature.

(3) Transfer the reaction solution to a beaker, add 37 mL distilled water, stir it evenly, let it sit at room temperature for 15 min, filter, and adjust the pH = 4~5 with 15% hydrochloric acid. Let the solid particles precipitate, then filter and wash with a small amount of cold water. Once crude phenytoin is obtained, dry and weigh it up. Finally, calculate the yield and measure the melting point.

4. Preparation of phenytoin sodium

(1) Equip the reaction apparatus.

(2) Add 1 g phenytoin and 5 mL water into the 100 mL three-neck round-bottom flask and heat to 40 ℃. Add 5 mL sodium hydroxide solution (15%) slowly until the solid is completely dissolved. Next, add activated carbon and heat the solution to 60 ℃ for 10 minutes. Filter the hot solution by vacuum filtration, stand it at room temperature for 20 minutes, and cool down with ice water. Solid particles will precipitate.

(3) Filter the solid precipitate and wash it with a small amount of ice water. Now, sodium phenytoin is obtained. Dry the product under an infrared lamp. Weigh the pure product, measure the melting point and calculate the yield.

(4) Send the final product to the place where the teachers designated.

V Experimental Results

1. Yield

(1) Calculate the theoretical production of phenytoin sodium

$$\text{Benzaldehyde} \longrightarrow \text{Phenytoin sodium}$$
$$M_w = 106.12 \text{ g/mol} \longrightarrow M_w = 274.25 \text{ g/mol}$$
$$0.098 \text{ mol} \longrightarrow 0.049 \text{ mol}$$

Theoretical production $= 0.049 \text{ mol} \times 274.25 \text{ g/mol} = 13.44 \text{ g}$

(2) Calculate the percent yield of phenytoin sodium

$$\text{Yield} = \frac{\text{Practical production}}{\text{Theoretical production}} \times 100\% = \frac{(\quad)}{13.44 \text{ g}} \times 100\% = (\quad)\%$$

2. Appearance and melting point of product

A. Appearance: _____ ;

B. m. p. :

    Theoretical value: 292~299 ℃

    Practical value: _____ .

3. Analysis of experimental results

_____

_____

_____

_____

_____

_____

_____

VI Notes

1. Benzaldehyde used in benzoin preparation needs to be newly distilled.

2. When 1,2-diphenylethylene ketone is prepared, the reaction system should be mildly boiling.

3. The control of reaction temperature in each step is important.

4. The whole reaction takes place in a sequence whereby the product of the one step will be used in the next step. So, the amount of each reagent used should be calculated proportionally.

VII Determination of Product Content

Chromatographic conditions: using octadecylsilane bonded silica gel as the filler. Using 0.05 mol/L ammonium dihydrogen phosphate (pH adjusted to 2.5 with phosphoric acid)-acetonitrile methanol (45 : 30 : 20) as the mobile phase. The flow rate is 1.5 mL per minute. The detection wavelength is 220 nm. The injection volume is 20 μL.

Measurement method: High-performance liquid chromatography method. Precisely weigh the test sample and reference solution, inject them into the liquid chromatograph separately, and record the chromatogram. Calculate based on peak area using the external standard method. (Chinese Pharmacopoeia 2020 Edition)

Ⅷ Discussion Questions

1. In terms of structure, what is the mechanism of benzoin condensation catalyzed by Vitamin B_1?

2. Can benzoin be oxidized with concentrated nitric acid in the preparation of 1,2-diphenylethylene ketone?

3. In terms of structure, explain the reaction mechanism for the formation of phenytoin.

(By Saiyang Zhang)

实验十三

苯妥英钠的合成

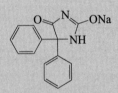

Ⅰ 目的与要求

    1. 掌握安息香缩合反应、氧化反应、重排反应的原理和操作要求。

    2. 了解苯妥英钠与靶标的作用方式。

Ⅱ 实验原理

1. 主要反应物和产物的物理常数

名称	结构式 CAS 号	分子式 分子量	沸点或熔点/℃	溶解度
苯甲醛	CHO 100-52-7	C_7H_6O 106.12	b. p. 179	水：<0.01 g/100 mL
安息香	OH O 119-53-9	$C_{14}H_{12}O_2$ 212.24	m. p. 134～138	不溶于水,微溶于醚类,溶于醇
1,2-二苯乙二酮	O O 579-07-7	$C_9H_8O_2$ 210.23	m. p. 95～96	溶于乙醇、乙醚、丙酮、苯、氯仿等有机溶剂,不溶于水

名称	结构式 CAS 号	分子式 分子量	沸点或熔点/℃	溶解度
苯妥英	57-41-0	$C_{15}H_{12}N_2O_2$ 252.27	m. p. 293～295	水：<0.01 g/100 mL，溶于 DMSO
苯妥英钠	630-93-3	$C_{15}H_{11}NaO_2$ 274.25	m. p. 292～299	易溶于水，溶于乙醇，不溶于氯仿
维生素 B_1	67-03-8	$C_{12}H_{16}N_4OS \cdot HCl$ 337.27	m. p. 245～250	极易溶于水，微溶于乙醇，不溶于乙醚、苯、氯仿和丙酮
六水合三氯化铁	$FeCl_3 \cdot 6H_2O$ 10025-77-1	$FeCl_3 \cdot 6H_2O$ 270.30	m. p. 37	易溶于水
尿素	NH_2CONH_2 57-13-6	CH_4N_2O 60.06	m. p. 132.7	溶于水、甲醇、甲醛、乙醇、液氨和醇，微溶于乙醚、氯仿、苯

2. 合成路线

苯甲醛在维生素 B_1 催化下，发生安息香缩合生成安息香；然后，氧化生成1,2-二苯乙二酮。随后，在碱性条件下，与尿素缩合并重排生成苯妥英。最后，经成盐反应得到苯妥英钠。

安全提示：苯甲醛对眼睛、呼吸道黏膜有一定的刺激作用。

3. 知识点

安息香缩合反应，氧化反应，重排反应，反应机理。

Ⅲ 实验装置和原料

1. 实验装置

反应装置由磁力搅拌器、三口烧瓶、回流冷凝管和温度计组成。

2. 原料

合成步骤	原料			
	名称	用量	试剂级别	用途
安息香	苯甲醛	10 mL(0.098 mol)	化学纯	反应物
	维生素 B_1	1.75 g(0.005 mol)	化学纯(60 %)	催化剂
	95 %乙醇	15 mL	—	溶剂
	2 mol/L NaOH	5 mL	—	催化剂
	蒸馏水	适量	—	溶剂
1,2-二苯乙二酮	安息香	2.12 g (0.010 mol)	自制	反应物
	六水合三氯化铁	9.0 g (0.033 mol)	化学纯	氧化剂
	冰醋酸	10 mL	化学纯	溶剂
	95 %乙醇	适量	化学纯	溶剂
	蒸馏水	适量	—	溶剂
	乙醚	适量	化学纯	溶剂
苯妥英	1,2-二苯乙二酮	1 g	自制	反应物
	尿素	0.57 g (0.0095 mol)	化学纯	反应物
	15 %NaOH	3.1 mL	自制	催化剂
	95 %乙醇	5 mL	化学纯	溶剂
	15 %盐酸	适量	—	中和反应
	蒸馏水	37 mL	—	溶剂
苯妥英钠	苯妥英	1 g	自制	反应物
	15 %氢氧化钠	5 mL	自制	反应物
	活性炭	适量	化学纯	脱色剂
	蒸馏水	5 mL	—	溶剂

Ⅳ 实验操作

1. 安息香合成

（1）搭建反应装置。

（2）在 50 mL 三口烧瓶中，加入 1.75 g 维生素 B_1、4 mL 蒸馏水，搅拌溶解，向上述溶液中加入 95 %乙醇，逐滴加入 2 mol/L 氢氧化钠水溶液。滴加完毕，室温搅拌 5 min，加入 10 mL 苯甲醛，搅拌均匀后，室温放置 1 周。

（3）将以上体系抽滤，滤饼用少量冷水洗涤，烘干，称重，计算收率，测熔点。

2. 1,2-二苯乙二酮合成

（1）搭建反应装置。

（2）在 100 mL 三口烧瓶中，加入 2.12 g 安息香、9.0 g 六水合三氯化铁和

5 mL 水，搅拌均匀后，加入 10 mL 冰醋酸，升温至回流反应 1 h。然后加入 50 mL 水，继续加热回流 5 min。

（3）将反应体系冷却至室温，析出固体，抽滤，得到的滤饼即为 1,2-二苯乙酮粗品。

（4）把粗品用 12 mL 乙醇重结晶，抽滤，用少量冷的乙醇和乙醚混合溶液洗涤滤饼，干燥，称重，计算收率。测熔点。

3. 苯妥英合成

（1）搭建反应装置。

（2）在 100 mL 三口烧瓶中，加入 1 g 1,2-二苯乙二酮、0.57 g 尿素、15％氢氧化钠和 5 mL 95％乙醇，升温至回流反应 2 h，降温至室温。

（3）将反应液转移至烧杯，加入蒸馏水，搅拌均匀，室温放置 15 min，抽滤。滤液用 15％的盐酸调节 pH 值为 4～5。析出固体，抽滤，少量冷水洗涤滤饼，得到苯妥英粗品，干燥，称重，计算收率。测熔点。

4. 苯妥英钠合成

（1）搭建反应装置。

（2）在 100 mL 三口烧瓶中，加入 1 g 苯妥英和 5 mL 水，升温至 40 ℃，缓慢加入 15％氢氧化钠水溶液 5 mL 直至固体完全溶解。加入活性炭，升温至 60 ℃并保温 10 min。热过滤，室温放置 20 min 后，冰水冷却。析出固体。

（3）过滤，少量冷水洗涤滤饼，真空干燥，得到苯妥英钠。称重，计算收率，测熔点。

（4）将产物送到指导教师指定的产品回收处。

V 实验结果

1. 收率

（1）计算苯妥英钠的理论产量

$$苯甲醛————苯妥英钠$$
$$M_w = 106.12 \text{ g/mol} ————M_w = 274.25 \text{ g/mol}$$
$$0.098 \text{ mol} ————0.049 \text{ mol}$$
$$理论产量 = 0.049 \text{ mol} \times 274.25 \text{ g/mol} = 13.44 \text{ g}$$

（2）计算苯妥英钠的收率

$$收率 = \frac{产品实际产量}{产品理论产量} \times 100\% = \frac{(\qquad)}{13.44 \text{ g}} \times 100\% = (\qquad)\%$$

2. 产品外观与熔点

A. 外观：_____；

B. 熔点：

　　理论值：292～299 ℃

　　实测值：_____。

3. 实验结果分析

_____

_____

_____

_____

VI 注意事项

1. 安息香制备所用的苯甲醛需要为新蒸馏过的。
2. 制备 1,2-二苯乙二酮时，反应体系应为温和沸腾状态。
3. 各个步骤中的反应温度控制是重要的因素。
4. 整个反应是接着上一步反应进行的，所用试剂的量需要按照比例计算后使用。

VII 产物的含量测定

色谱条件：以十八烷基硅烷键合硅胶为填充剂；以 0.05 mol/L 磷酸二氢铵（用磷酸调节 pH 值至 2.5）-乙腈-甲醇（45：30：20）为流动相；流速为每分钟 1.5 mL；检测波长为 220 nm；进样体积 20 μL。

测定法：采用高效液相色谱法。精密量取供试品与对照品溶液，分别注入液相色谱仪，记录色谱图。按照外标法以峰面积计算。（《中华人民共和国药典（2020 年版）》）

VIII 思考题

1. 用结构式表示，维生素 B_1 催化的安息香缩合反应机理。
2. 制备 1,2-二苯乙二酮时，能用浓硝酸氧化安息香吗？
3. 用结构式表示，生成苯妥英这一步反应的反应机理。

（张赛扬）

Experiment 14

Synthesis of Neostigmine Bromide

Background

Neostigmine bromide is a reversible anti-cholinesterase drug used for the treatment of myasthenia gravis, intestinal paralysis and urinary retention after abdominal surgery. The chemical structure of neostigmine bromide is shown in Fig. 14-1.

Fig. 14-1　Structure of Neostigmine Bromide

The mechanism of action of Neostigmine bromide

Ⅰ　Purposes and Requirements

1. To master the reaction principle and experimental operations of N-alkylation reaction, esterification reaction principle and operation requirements.

2. To understand the interaction between neostigmine bromide and target.

Ⅱ　Principle of the Reaction

1. Physical data of the main reactants and product

Name	Structure CAS No.	Formula M. Wt	b. p. or m. p. /℃	Solubility
m-Aminophenol	591-27-5	C_6H_7NO 109.05	m. p. 121	Slightly soluble in water, ethanol, and ether
Dimethyl sulfate	77-78-1	$C_2H_6O_4S$ 126.13	b. p. 188(Decompose)	Soluble in ethanol, ether, dioxane, acetone, and aromatic hydrocarbons; decomposition in water

Name	Structure CAS No.	Formula M. Wt	b. p. or m. p. /°C	Solubility
m-Dimethylaminophenol	N(CH$_3$)$_2$ ... OH 99-07-0	C$_8$H$_{11}$NO 137. 18	m. p. 82~84	Soluble in ethanol, ether, acetone, benzene, alkali, and inorganic acid; almost insoluble in water
Dimethylcarbamoyl chloride	Cl—C—N(CH$_3$)$_2$ (O) 79-44-7	C$_3$H$_6$ClNO 107. 54	b. p. 167~168	Decompose in water; soluble in ether, benzene, and carbon disulfide
m-dimethylaminophenyl dimethylcarbamate (Neostigmine)	N(CH$_3$)$_2$ ... O—C—N(CH$_3$)$_2$ (O) 16088-19-0	C$_{11}$H$_{16}$N$_2$O$_2$ 208. 26	b. p. 313. 6	Soluble in acetone and ethanol
Neostigmine bromide	N$^+$(CH$_3$)$_3$ · Br$^-$ ... O—C—N(CH$_3$)$_2$ (O) 114-80-7	C$_{12}$H$_{19}$BrN$_2$O$_2$ 303. 2	m. p. 175~177	Well soluble in water; soluble in ethanol and chloroform; insoluble in ether
Triethylamine	N(CH$_2$CH$_3$)$_3$ 121-44-8	C$_6$H$_{15}$N 101. 19	b. p. 89. 5	—
Pyridine	(pyridine ring) N 110-86-1	C$_5$H$_5$N 79. 1	m. p. 96~98	Soluble in water and common organic solvents
Toluene	CH$_3$ (benzene ring) 108-88-3	C$_7$H$_8$ 92. 14	b. p. 110	Insoluble in water, soluble in most organic solvents such as benzene, alcohol, and ether
Methyl bromide	CH$_3$Br 74-83-9	CH$_3$Br 94. 94	b. p. 3. 6	Insoluble in water; soluble in most organic solvents such as ethanol, ether, chloroform, benzene, etc.

2. Synthetic route

$$\text{m-Aminophenol} \xrightarrow[]{(CH_3)_2SO_4,\ PhCH_3} \text{3-Dimethylaminophenol} \xrightarrow[PhCH_3,\ Et_3N]{Cl-C(O)-N(CH_3)_2}$$

m-Aminophenol   3-Dimethylaminophenol

$$\text{Neostigmine} \xrightarrow{\text{CH}_3\text{Br}} \text{Neostigmine bromide}$$

Neostigmine   Neostigmine bromide

m-Dimethylaminophenol is formed by *N*-alkylation of *m*-aminophenol and dimethyl sulfate, which is subsequently esterified with *N*, *N*-dimethylcarbamoyl chloride to produce neostigmine. And then, neostigmine bromide was synthesized by quaternary ammoniation with methyl bromide.

Safety Tips: Dimethyl sulfate has a strong irritating effect on eyes and upper respiratory tract, and a strong corrosive effect on the skin.

N, *N*-dimethylcarbamoyl chloride has strong irritation to the eyes, skin, mucosa and respiratory tract. It should be used in the fume hood.

3. Knowledge points

The *N*-alkylation reaction, esterification reaction, precautions for the use of acyl chloride and dimethyl sulfate.

N-alkylation reaction apparatus and salt formation apparatus

Ⅲ Experimental Equipment and Raw Materials

1. Experimental equipment

N-alkylation reaction apparatus is composed of a magnetic stirrer, a three-neck round-bottom flask, a spherical condenser tube, a thermometer, a constant pressure dropping funnel, and a drying tube.

Salt formation reaction apparatus is composed of a magnetic stirrer, a three-neck round-bottom flask, a spherical condenser tube, a gasing rubber tube, and a thermometer.

2. Raw materials

Synthetic product	Raw materials			
	Name	Quantity	Quality	Use
m-Dimethylami-nophenol	*m*-Aminophenol	22 g (0. 2 mol)	CP	Reactant
	Dimethyl sulfate	38. 8 mL (0. 4 mol)	CP	Reactant
	Toluene	50 mL	CP	Solvent
	Sodium carbonate	Proper amount	CP	Neutralization reaction
	Distilled water	Proper amount	—	Solvent
m-Dimethylami-nophenyl dimeth-ylcarbamate (Neostigmine)	*m*-Dimethylaminophenol	13. 7 g (0. 1 mol)	Product prepared	Reactant
	Dimethylcarbamoyl chloride	11. 8 g (0. 11 mol)	CP	Acylation reagent
	Triethylamine	20. 8 mL (0. 15 mol)	CP	Acid-binding agent
	Pyridine	1. 6 mL (0. 02 mol)	CP	Acid-binding agent
	Toluene	100 mL	CP	Solvent
	NaOH	Proper amount	CP	Neutralization reaction

Synthetic product	Raw materials			
	Name	Quantity	Quality	Use
m-Dimethylami-nophenyl dimeth-ylcarbamate (Neostigmine)	Distilled water	Proper amount	—	Solvent
	Silica Gel for Chromatography	5 g	CP	Adsorption impurity
	Anhydrous sodium sulfate	proper amount	CP	Dehydrant
Neostigmine bromide	Neostigmine	10. 4 g (0. 05 mol)	Product prepared	Reactant
	Methyl bromide	4. 1 mL (0. 075 mol)	CP	Reactant
	Acetone	20 mL	CP	Solvent
	Absolute ethanol	30 mL	CP	Solvent
	Activated carbon	0. 5 g	CP	Discolouring agent

IV Operations

1. Preparation of m -dimethylaminophenol

(1) Equip the N-alkylation reaction apparatus.

(2) Add 22 g m-aminophenol and 50 mL toluene into the 250 mL three-neck round-bottom flask, and dissolve it completely by stirring. Next, add 38. 8 mL dimethyl sulfate (treated with anhydrous sodium carbonate to pH = 5) dropwise within 30 minutes. Heat the solution to 75 ℃ for 3 h and cool down to room temperature.

(3) Separate the organic layer and adjust the pH to 9 with sodium carbonate solution. Separate the organic layer again and remove toluene by rotating evaporation. Distill the residues by vacuum distillation at 138~150 ℃/10 mmHg and collect the fraction. m-Dimethyl-aminophenol is obtained when the fraction is frozen. Dry the product under an infrared lamp and weigh it up. Calculate the yield and measure the melting point.

2. Preparation of neostigmine

(1) Equip the N-alkylation reaction apparatus.

(2) Add 13. 7 g m-Dimethylaminophenol, 20. 8 mL triethylamine, 1. 6 mL pyridine, and 100 mL toluene into the 250 mL three-neck round-bottom flask and stir it evenly. Add 7. 1 g N,N-dimethylcarbamoyl chloride dropwise at room temperature and heat to 45~50 ℃ for 3 h.

(3) Cool the reaction solution to room temperature, add 100 mL distilled water and stir evenly. Separate the organic layer, wash it with 10 % sodium hydroxide solution, and add anhydrous sodium sulfate to dry overnight.

(4) Remove the sodium sulfate by filtration. Add 5 g silica gel to the organic layer and stir it evenly. Remove the silica gel by filtration. Rotate the filtrate to remove the solvent. The residue is neostigmine. Dry the product under an infrared lamp and weigh it up. Calculate the yield and measure the melting point.

3. Preparation of neostigmine bromide

(1) Equip the salt formation reaction apparatus.

(2) Add 10.4 g neostigmine and 20 mL acetone into the 100 mL three-neck round-bottom flask and cool it to 5 ℃. Add 4.1 mL methane bromide and store at room temperature for 3 days. Crystals will be precipitated.

(3) The crude neostigmine bromide is obtained by filtration.

(4) Dissolve the crude product in anhydrous ethanol (30 mL), then reflux with 0.5 g activated carbon for 5 minutes. Filter the hot solution and cool it to room temperature. Precipitate the solids and filter. Wash the filter cake is with a small amount of cold ethanol to obtain pure bromo-neostigmine.

(5) Dry the product under infrared lamp and weigh it up. Calculate the yield and measure the melting point.

(6) Send the finished product to the place where the teachers designated.

Ⅴ Experimental Results

1. Yield

(1) Calculate the theoretical production of neostigmine bromide

$$m\text{-Aminophenol} \longrightarrow \text{Neostigmine bromide}$$
$$M_w = 109.05 \text{ g/mol} \longrightarrow M_w = 303.2 \text{ g/mol}$$
$$0.2 \text{ mol} \longrightarrow 0.2 \text{ mol}$$

Theoretical production $= 0.2 \text{ mol} \times 303.2 \text{ g/mol} = 60.64 \text{ g}$

(2) Calculate the percent yield of neostigmine bromide

$$\text{Yield} = \frac{\text{Practical production}}{\text{Theoretical production}} \times 100\% = \frac{(\qquad)}{60.64 \text{ g}} \times 100\% = (\qquad)\%$$

2. Appearance and melting point of product

Physical Identification

A. Appearance: _____ ;

B. m. p. :

Theoretical value: 175~177 ℃

Practical value: _____ .

3. Analysis of experimental results

_____

_____

_____

_____

_____

_____ .

Ⅵ Notes

1. The synthetic step of m-dimethylaminophenol is an anhydrous reaction. The reagents and instruments used need to be dried before use.

2. When neostigmine bromide is refined, if the product does not precipitate at room temperature, it should be placed in ice bath at 0 ℃.

3. The control of reaction temperature in each step is an important factor.

4. The whole reaction takes place in a sequence whereby the product of the one step will be used in the next step. So, the amount of each reagent used should be calculated proportionally.

Ⅶ Determination of Product Content

Titration method: Take about 0.2 g of this product, accurately weigh it, dissolve it in a mixed solution of 20 mL of glacial acetic acid and 5 mL of mercuric acetate test solution, add 1 drop of crystal violet indicator solution, titrate with perchloric acid titrant (0.1 mol/L) until the solution turns blue, and calibrate the titration results with a blank test. Each 1 mL of perchloric acid titrant (0.1 mol/L) is equivalent to 30.32 mg of neostigmine bromide. (Chinese Pharmacopoeia 2020 Edition)

Ⅷ Discussion Questions

1. In terms of structure, what substances can be used to replace triethylamine in the esterification reaction to produce neostigmine?

2. In terms of structure, explain the reaction mechanism for the formation of neostigmine.

(By Wen Li)

实验十四
溴新斯的明的合成

背景知识

溴新斯的明（Neostigmine bromide），是一种可逆性抗胆碱酯酶药，用于重症肌无力、腹部术后的肠麻痹和尿潴留等症，其化学结构见图 14-1。

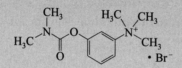

溴新斯的明作用机制

图 14-1　溴新斯的明化学结构

Ⅰ 目的与要求

1. 掌握 N-烷基化反应、酯化反应的合成原理和实验操作。
2. 了解溴新斯的明与靶标作用方式。

Ⅱ 实验原理

1. 主要反应物和产物的物理常数

名称	结构式 CAS 号	分子式 分子量	沸点或 熔点/℃	溶解度
间氨基苯酚	591-27-5	C_6H_7NO 109.05	m. p. 121	微溶于水、溶于醇、醚
硫酸二甲酯	77-78-1	$C_2H_6O_4S$ 126.13	b. p. 188（分解）	溶于乙醇、乙醚、二氧六环、丙酮和芳香烃类，遇水分解

名称	结构式 CAS 号	分子式 分子量	沸点或 熔点/℃	溶解度
间二甲氨基苯酚	N(CH$_3$)$_2$ [苯环] OH 99-07-0	C$_8$H$_{11}$NO 137.18	m. p. 82～84	溶于乙醇、乙醚、丙酮、苯、碱和无机酸,几乎不溶于水
N,N-二甲氨基甲酰氯	Cl—C(=O)—N(CH$_3$)$_2$ 79-44-7	C$_3$H$_6$ClNO 107.54	b. p. 167～168	遇水分解,溶于乙醚、苯和二硫化碳
新斯的明	N(CH$_3$)$_2$ [苯环] O—C(=O)—N(CH$_3$)$_2$ 16088-19-0	C$_{11}$H$_{16}$N$_2$O$_2$ 208.26	b. p. 313.6	溶于丙酮,乙醇
溴新斯的明	N$^+$(CH$_3$)$_3$·Br$^-$ [苯环] O—C(=O)—N(CH$_3$)$_2$ 114-80-7	C$_{12}$H$_{19}$BrN$_2$O$_2$ 303.2	m. p. 175～177	易溶于水,溶于乙醇、氯仿,不溶于乙醚
三乙胺	N(CH$_2$CH$_3$)$_3$ 121-44-8	C$_6$H$_{15}$N 101.19	b. p. 89.5	—
吡啶	[吡啶环] N 110-86-1	C$_5$H$_5$N 79.1	m. p. 96～98	可溶于水和常用有机溶剂
甲苯	CH$_3$ [苯环] 108-88-3	C$_7$H$_8$ 92.14	b. p. 110	不溶于水,可混溶于苯、醇、醚等多数有机溶剂
溴甲烷	CH$_3$Br 74-83-9	CH$_3$Br 94.94	b. p. 3.6	不溶于水,溶于乙醇、乙醚、氯仿、苯等多数有机溶剂

2. 合成路线

间氨基苯酚 (NH$_2$，OH苯环) →[(CH$_3$)$_2$SO$_4$, PhCH$_3$] 间二甲氨基苯酚 (N(CH$_3$)$_2$，OH苯环) →[Cl—C(=O)—N(CH$_3$)$_2$；PhCH$_3$, Et$_3$N]

新斯的明 $\xrightarrow{\text{CH}_3\text{Br}}$ 溴新斯的明

间氨基苯酚与硫酸二甲酯发生 N-烷基化反应生成间二甲氨基苯酚，然后与 N,N-二甲氨基甲酰氯发生酯化反应生成新斯的明，随后，与溴甲烷成季铵盐得到溴新斯的明。

安全提示：硫酸二甲酯对眼、上呼吸道有强烈刺激作用，对皮肤有强腐蚀作用。

N,N-二甲氨基甲酰氯对眼睛、皮肤黏膜和呼吸道有强烈的刺激作用。故该试剂应在通风橱中使用。

Ⅲ 实验装置和原料

1. 实验装置

N-烷基化反应装置由磁力搅拌器、三口烧瓶、回流冷凝管、温度计、滴液漏斗和干燥管组成。

成盐反应装置由磁力搅拌器、三口烧瓶、回流冷凝管、导气管和温度计组成。

N-烷基化反应装置和成盐反应装置

2. 原料

合成产物	原料			
	名称	用量	试剂级别	用途
间二甲氨基苯酚	间氨基苯酚	22 g(0.2 mol)	化学纯	反应物
	硫酸二甲酯	38.8 mL(0.4 mol)	化学纯	反应物
	甲苯	50 mL	化学纯	溶剂
	碳酸钠	适量	化学纯	中和酸
	蒸馏水	适量	—	溶剂
新斯的明	间二甲氨基苯酚	13.7 g(0.1 mol)	自制	反应物
	N,N-二甲氨基甲酰氯	11.8 g(0.11 mol)	化学纯	酰化试剂
	三乙胺	20.8 mL(0.15 mol)	化学纯	缚酸剂
新斯的明	吡啶	1.6 mL(0.02 mol)	化学纯	缚酸剂
	甲苯	100 mL	化学纯	溶剂
	氢氧化钠	适量	化学纯	中和酸
	蒸馏水	适量	—	溶剂
	色谱用硅胶	5 g	化学纯	吸附杂质
	无水硫酸钠	适量	化学纯	干燥除水
溴新斯的明	新斯的明	10.4 g(0.05 mol)	自制	反应物
	溴甲烷	4.1 mL(0.075 mol)	化学纯	反应物
	丙酮	20 mL	化学纯	溶剂
	无水乙醇	30 mL	化学纯	溶剂
	活性炭	0.5 g	化学纯	脱色剂

Ⅳ 实验操作

1. 间二甲氨基苯酚合成

（1）搭建 *N*-烷基化反应装置。

（2）在 250 mL 三口烧瓶中，加入 22 g 间氨基苯酚和 50 mL 甲苯，搅拌溶解，在 30 min 内逐滴加入 38.8 mL 硫酸二甲酯（用无水碳酸钠处理至 pH 值为 5）。滴加完毕，升温至 75 ℃反应 3 h。冷却至室温。

（3）分取有机层，加碳酸钠水溶液调节 pH＝9，再次分取有机层，旋转蒸发除去甲苯，残留物减压蒸馏，收集 138～150 ℃/10 mmHg 的馏分，固化后得到间二甲氨基苯酚，称重，计算收率，测熔点。

2. 新斯的明合成

（1）搭建 *N*-烷基化反应装置。

（2）在 250 mL 三口烧瓶中，加入 13.7 g 间二甲氨基苯酚、20.8 mL 三乙胺、1.6 mL 吡啶和 100 mL 甲苯，搅拌均匀后，室温滴加 7.1 g *N*,*N*-二甲氨基甲酰氯，升温至 45～50 ℃反应 3 h。

（3）反应体系冷却至室温，加入蒸馏水 100 mL，搅拌均匀后，分取有机层，10 ％氢氧化钠溶液洗涤，加入无水硫酸钠干燥过夜。

（4）过滤除去硫酸钠，有机层加入层析用硅胶 5 g 搅拌均匀，过滤，滤液旋蒸除去溶剂，残留物为新斯的明。称重，计算收率。

3. 溴新斯的明合成

（1）搭建成盐反应装置。

（2）在 100 mL 三口烧瓶中，加入 10.4 g 新斯的明和 20 mL 丙酮，冷却至 5 ℃后，通入 4.1 mL 溴甲烷，室温放置 3 天。析出晶体。

（3）过滤，得到溴新斯的明粗品。

（4）将粗品用 30 mL 无水乙醇加热溶解，加入活性炭回流 5 min，过滤，冷却至室温，析出固体，抽滤，少量冷乙醇洗涤滤饼，得到溴新斯的明精制品。

（5）烘干纯品，称重，计算收率，测熔点。

（6）将产物送到指导教师指定的产品回收处。

Ⅴ 实验结果

1. 收率

（1）计算溴新斯的明的理论产量

$$间氨基苯酚————溴新斯的明$$

$$M_w—109.05 \text{ g/mol} \qquad M_w＝303.2 \text{ g/mol}$$

$$0.2 \text{ mol}————0.2 \text{ mol}$$

$$理论产量＝0.2 \text{ mol}×303.2 \text{ g/mol}＝60.64 \text{ g}$$

（2）计算溴新斯的明的收率

$$收率＝\frac{产品实际产量}{产品理论产量}×100 ％＝\frac{(\qquad)}{60.64 \text{ g}}×100 ％＝(\qquad) ％$$

2. 产品外观与熔点

A. 外观：_____；

B. 熔点：

理论值：175～177 ℃；

实测值：_____。

3. 实验结果分析

_____

_____

_____

_____

_____

_____。

Ⅵ 注意事项

1. 间二甲氨基苯酚合成步骤为无水反应，所用试剂和仪器需要干燥后使用。

2. 溴新斯的明精制时，若室温不析出产品，冰浴 0 ℃放置。

3. 各步骤反应温度控制是重要的因素。

4. 整个反应是接着上一步反应进行的，所用试剂的量需要按照比例计算后使用。

Ⅶ 产物的含量测定

滴定法：取本品约 0.2 g，精密称定，加冰醋酸 20 mL 与醋酸汞试液 5 mL 使溶解，加结晶紫指示液 1 滴，用高氯酸滴定液（0.1 mol/L）滴定至溶液显蓝色，并将滴定的结果用空白试验校正，每 1 mL 高氯酸滴定液（0.1 mol/L）相当于 30.32 mg 的溴新斯的明。（《中华人民共和国药典（2020 年版）》）

Ⅷ 思考题

1. 用结构式表示，酯化反应生成新斯的明时，可用什么物质取代三乙胺？

2. 用结构式表示，生成新斯的明这一步反应的反应机理。

（李雯）

Experiment 15

Synthesis of Boceprevir

Background

Boceprevir is a hepatitis C treatment drug, marketed under the brand name victrelis, and was approved for sale in the United States in 2011. The chemical structure of Boceprevir is shown in Fig. 15-1.

Fig. 15-1 Chemical structure of Boceprevir

The mechanism of action of Boceprevir

Ⅰ Purposes and Requirements

1. To master the principles and experimental operations of amidation, hydrolysis, and oxidation reactions.

2. To understand the mode of action of Boceprevir and its target.

Ⅱ Principle of the Reaction

1. Physical data of the main reactants and product

Name	Structure CAS No.	Formula M. Wt	b. p. or m. p. / ℃	Solubility
(S)-2-[3-(tert-Butyl) ureido]-3,3-dimethylbutyric acid(compound **2**)	101968-85-8	$C_{11}H_{22}N_2O_3$ 230.30	m. p. 182	—

Name	Structure CAS No.	Formula M. Wt	b. p. or m. p. / ℃	Solubility
(1*R*,2*S*,5*S*)-Methyl 6,6-dimethyl-3-azabicyclo[3.1.0]hexane-2-carboxylate hydrochloride (compound **3**)	565456-77-1	$C_9H_{16}ClNO_2$ 205.68	—	—
1-Ethyl-3-(3-dimethylaminopropyl)carbodiimide hydrochloride (EDC·HCl)	25952-53-8	$C_8H_{18}ClN_3$ 191.70	m. p. 110~115	Soluble in water and ethanol
4-Methylmorpholine (NMM)	109-02-4	$C_5H_{11}NO$ 101.15	b. p. 115.4	Soluble in water
Sodium hydroxide	NaOH 1310-73-2	NaOH 40.00	m. p. 318.4	Soluble in water, ethanol, and glycerol; insoluble in ether, acetone
HOBt	2592-95-2	$C_6H_5N_3O$ 135.12	m. p. 156~159	Soluble in DMSO (little amount), methanol (little amount)
3-Amino-4-cyclobutyl-2-hydroxybutanamide hydrochloride (compound **6**)	394735-23-0	$C_8H_{17}ClN_2O_2$ 208.69	m. p. 196~200	Soluble in DMSO (little amount), methanol (little amount)
Dess-Martin oxidizer	87413-09-0	$C_{13}H_{13}IO_8$ 424.14	m. p. 130~133	Slightly soluble in CH_2Cl_2, $CHCl_3$, MeCN, and THF
Boceprevir	394730-60-0	$C_{27}H_{45}N_5O_5$ 519.68	m. p. 107(decompose)	DMSO:16.67~100 mg/mL H_2O:<0.1 mg/mL Ethanol:~100 mg/mL

2. Synthetic route

The synthesis of Boceprevir (Compound **1**) is carried out using tert leucine urea (Compound **2**) and dimethylcyclopropylproline analogue (Compound **3**) as raw materials, with EDC • HCl as the condensing agent. Intermediate compound **4** is obtained through an amidation reaction, and compound **5** is obtained after hydrolysis of the intermediate. Subsequently, the obtained compound **5** undergoes an amidation reaction with racemic β-aminoamide (compound **6**) to obtain compound **7**. Finally, compound **7** is treated with Dess-Martin oxidizer to obtain the target compound **1**.

Safety Tips: Dess-Martin oxidizer (DMP) may explode upon impact or heating to > 130 ℃. All operations related to DMP must be completed under cooling conditions.

3. Knowledge points

Acylation reaction, hydrolysis reaction, oxidation reaction, EDC • HCl, Dess-Martin oxidizer.

Ⅲ Experimental Equipments and Raw Materials

1. Experimental equipment

The acylation apparatus is composed of a magnetic stirrer, an ice-water

The acylation apparatus

bath, a three-necked round-bottom flask, a reflux condenser, and a thermometer.

2. Raw materials

Synthetic product	Raw materials			
	Name	Quantity	Quality	Use
Compound 4	(S)-2-[3-(Tert butyl)ureido]-3,3-dimethylbutyric acid	10.08 g (0.0438 mol)	—	Reactant
	(1R,2S,5S)-6,6-Dimethyl-3-azabicyclo[3.1.0]hexane-2-carboxylic acid methyl ester hydrochloride	9 g (0.0438 mol)	—	Reactant
	N,N-Dimethylformamide	45 mL	AR	Solvent
	Toluene	45 mL	AR	Solvent
	1-Ethyl-3-(3-dimethylaminopropyl) carbodiimide hydrochloride(EDC · HCl)	10.89 g (0.0567 mol)	AR	Reactant
	4-Methylmorpholine(NMM)	11.07 g (0.1092 mol)	AR	Base
	Distilled water	135 mL	—	Solvent
	1 mol/L Hydrochloric acid solution	45 mL	Prepared solution	Adjust pH value
	10% Sodium bicarbonate solution	45 mL	Prepared solution	Adjust pH value
Compound 5	Compound 4	5 g (0.0131 mol)	—	Reactant
	Toluene	50 mL	AR	Solvent
	Methanol	5 mL	AR	Solvent
	47% Sodium hydroxide solution	1.58 mL	Prepared solution	Base
	Distilled water	25 mL	—	Solvent
	1 mol/L Hydrochloric acid solution	25 mL	Prepared solution	Adjust pH value
	Ethyl Acetate	50 mL	AR	Solvent
	Methyl tert-butyl ether	25 mL	AR	Solvent
Compound 7	Compound 5	4 g (0.0108 mol)	—	Reactant
	3-Amino-4-cyclobutyl-2-hydroxybutanamide hydrochloride	2.5 g (0.0119 mol)	—	Reactant
	Ethyl Acetate	32 mL	AR	Solvent
	N,N-Dimethylformamide	8 mL	AR	Solvent
	1-Ethyl-3-(3-dimethylaminopropyl) carbodiimide hydrochloride(EDC · HCl)	2.5 g (0.013 mol)	AR	Reactant
	1-Hydroxybenzotriazole	0.3 g (0.0022 mol)	AR	Racemization inhibitor
	4-Methylmorpholine (NMM)	2.75 g (0.0271 mol)	AR	Base
	Distilled water	30 mL	—	Solvent
	1 mol/L hydrochloric acid solution	20 mL	Prepared solution	Adjust pH value
	10% Sodium bicarbonate solution	20 mL	Prepared solution	Adjust pH value
	n-Heptane	24 mL	AR	Solvent

Synthetic product	Raw materials			
	Name	Quantity	Quality	Use
Boceprevir (Compound **1**)	Compound **7**	2 g (0.0038 mol)	—	Reactant
	Ethyl Acetate	35 mL	AR	Solvent
	Dess-Martin Periodinane	2.6 g (0.0061 mol)	AR	Oxidant
	Methyl tert-butyl ether	10 mL	AR	Solvent
	40% Sodium bisulfite solution	Appropriate amount	—	Antioxidant
	n-Heptane	24 mL	AR	Solvent

Ⅳ Operations

1. Preparation of compound 4

(1) Equip the acylation apparatus.

(2) Place the dry 100 mL three-necked flask in an ice-water bath at 0~10 ℃. While stirring, add 10.08 g of compound **2**, 9 g of compound **3**, and 90 mL of DMF-toluene mixed solution (volume ratio is 1 : 1). Then, add 10.89 g of EDC • HCl and 11.07 g of 4-methylmorpholine to the mixture.

(3) Stir the reaction mixture at 0~10 ℃ for 4~5 h.

(4) After the reaction is complete, slowly add 90 mL of water at 0~10 ℃. Separate the organic layer and wash it sequentially with 45 mL of 1 mol/L HCl solution, 45 mL of 10% $NaHCO_3$ solution, 45 mL of water, and 45 mL of saline solution. Dry with anhydrous sodium sulfate.

(5) Filter, rotary evaporate to remove solvent, obtain white solid, dry, and weigh it.

2. Preparation of compound 5

(1) Equip the acylation apparatus.

(2) Place the 100 mL three-necked flask in an ice-water bath at 0~10 ℃. While stirring, add 50 mL of toluene, 5 g of compound **4**, 5 mL of methanol, and 1.58 mL of 47% sodium hydroxide solution.

(3) After adding, slowly raise the temperature to 25~30 ℃ and stir the reactants at this temperature for 3~4 h.

(4) After the reaction is complete, add 25 mL of water to the reaction mixture and separate the water layer.

(5) Acid the aqueous layer with 25 mL of 1 mol/L HCl solution to pH=2, and extract the product with ethyl acetate (2×25 mL). Dry it.

(6) Concentrate the organic layer by vacuum evaporation to 80%, and add pre-cooled 25 mL of methyl tert butyl ether at 5~10 ℃.

(7) Stir the material at 5~10 ℃ for 2~3 h.

(8) Filter to obtain a white solid, dry, and weigh it.

3. Preparation of compound 7

(1) Equip the acylation apparatus.

(2) Place the 100 mL three-necked flask in an ice-water bath at $0\sim10$ ℃. While stirring, add 4 g of compound **5**, 2.50 g of 3-amino-4-cyclobutyl-2-hydroxybutanamide hydrochloride (compound **6**), 32 mL of ethyl acetate, and 8 mL of DMF, stir and dissolve. Then, add 2.5 g EDC・HCl, 0.3 g HOBt, and 2.75 g 4-methylmorpholine.

(3) Stir the reaction mixture at $0\sim10$ ℃ for $5\sim6$ h.

(4) After the reaction is complete, add 30 mL of water at $0\sim10$ ℃. Separate the organic layer and wash it with 20 mL of 1 mol/L HCl solution, followed by 20 mL of 10% NaHCO$_3$ solution. Separate the organic layer and dry it.

(5) Concentrate the organic layer by vacuum evaporation to 80%, and add pre-cooled 24 mL of heptane at $0\sim10$ ℃.

(6) Filter to obtain a white to off-white solid, dry, and weigh it.

4. Preparation of Boceprevir (Compound 1)

(1) Equip the acylation apparatus.

(2) Place the 100 mL three-necked flask in an ice-water bath at $0\sim10$ ℃. While stirring, add 2 g of compound **7** and 20 mL of ethyl acetate. Then, add 2.6 g of Dess-Martin oxidizer in three equal intervals of 45 min.

(3) Stir the reaction mixture at $12\sim18$ ℃ for 3 h.

(4) After the reaction is complete, filter the reactants through diatomaceous earth under vacuum. Wash the filtrate with water and add 40% sodium bisulfite solution to the organic layer.

(5) Stir the solution at $25\sim30$ ℃ for $12\sim15$ h. Separate the organic layer and dry it.

(6) Concentrate the organic layer by vacuum evaporation to 80%, and add 8 mL of cyclohexane. Stir the mixture at $25\sim30$ ℃ for 1 h.

(7) Filter to obtain sulfite adduct.

(8) Dissolve the sulfite adduct in a mixed solvent of 5 mL of water and 10 mL of ethyl acetate, cool to $0\sim3$ ℃, and stir for $10\sim15$ min.

(9) Separate the water layer. Wash the water layer with 5 mL of ethyl acetate at $0\sim3$ ℃. Add 10 mL of methyl tert butyl ether to the water layer and stir the reaction mixture at $25\sim30$ ℃ for $2\sim3$ h. Separate the organic layer and dry it.

(10) Concentrate the organic layer by vacuum evaporation to 80%, and add pre-cooled 24 mL of heptane at $0\sim5$ ℃. Stir at this temperature for $30\sim45$ min.

(11) Filter to obtain a white solid, dry and weigh it, calculate the yield, and measure the melting point.

(12) Send the final product to the place where the teachers designated.

V Experimental Results

1. Yield

(1) Calculate the theoretical production of Boceprevir

$$\text{Compound } \textbf{2} \text{ ———— Boceprevir}$$
$$M_{\text{w}}=230.30 \text{ g/mol} \text{————} M_{\text{w}}=519.68 \text{ g/mol}$$

$$0.0438 \text{ mol} \text{———} 0.0438 \text{ mol}$$

Theoretical production$=0.0438 \text{ mol} \times 519.68 \text{ g/mol} = 22.76 \text{ g}$

(2) Calculate the percent yield of Boceprevir

$$\text{Yield} = \frac{\text{Practical production}}{\text{Theoretical production}} \times 100\% = \frac{(\quad)}{22.76 \text{ g}} \times 100\% = (\quad) \%$$

2. Appearance and melting point of product

A. Appearance: _____ ;

B. m. p. :

　Theoretical value: 107 ℃ (decompose);

　Practical value: _____ .

3. Analysis of experimental results

_____

_____

_____

_____

Ⅵ Notes

1. To avoid the generation of by-products, the reaction should be slowly heated up.

2. All experimental operations should be carried out in accordance with the specifications.

3. The entire reaction proceeds from the previous step, and the amount of each reagent used needs to be calculated proportionally before use.

Ⅶ Determination of Product Content

Chromatographic conditions: Poroshell, 100 mm × 4.6 mm, 2.7 μm; flow: 0.8 mL/min; buffer: 0.01 mol/L NaH_2PO_4 in water, pH adjusted to 7.0 with NaOH; eluent A: buffer and methanol in the ratio of 90 : 10, B: methanol and water in the ratio of 80 : 20. Gradient is that 0 min: 70% A, 30% B; 10 min: 40% A, 60% B; 15 min: 25% A, 75% B; 35 min: 10% A, 90% B; 41 min: 70% A, 30% B; 50 min: 70% A, 30% B. Column temperature: 40 ℃; UV detection at 220 nm.

Measurement method: High-performance liquid chromatography method. Accurately weigh the test sample, inject it into the liquid chromatograph, and record the chromatogram. Calculate the peak area. [Bhalerao DS, et al. Organic Process Research & Development, 2015, 19 (11): 1559-1567]

Ⅷ Discussion Questions

1. What is the principle of the reaction between compounds 2 and 3 in this experiment?

2. In terms of structure, what other alternatives can be used to represent the coupling reagent EDC · HCl?

(By Peng Sang)

▲

实验十五

波普瑞韦的合成

▼

波普瑞韦的
作用机制

背景知识

波普瑞韦（Boceprevir）是丙型肝炎治疗药物，其商品名为 victrelis，于 2011 年在美国获批准上市。波普瑞韦的化学结构如图 15-1 所示。

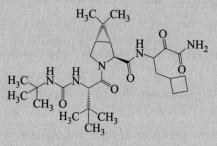

图 15-1　波普瑞韦的化学结构

Ⅰ　目的与要求

1. 掌握酰胺化、水解和氧化反应的原理及实验操作。
2. 了解波普瑞韦与靶标的作用方式。

Ⅱ　实验原理

1. 主要反应物和产物的物理常数

名称	结构式 CAS 号	分子式 分子量	沸点或 熔点/℃	溶解性
(S)-2-(3-(叔丁基)脲基)-3,3-二甲基丁酸（化合物 **2**）	101968-85-8	$C_{11}H_{22}N_2O_3$ 230.30	m. p. 182	—
(1R,2S,5S)-6,6-二甲基-3-氮杂双环[3.1.0]己烷-2-羧酸甲酯盐酸盐（化合物 **3**）	565456-77-1	$C_9H_{16}ClNO_2$ 205.68	—	—

名称	结构式 CAS 号	分子式 分子量	沸点或 熔点/℃	溶解性
1-乙基-3-(3-二甲基氨基丙基)碳酰二亚胺盐酸盐(EDC·HCl)	25952-53-8	$C_8H_{18}ClN_3$ 191.70	m. p. 110~115	溶于水和乙醇
N-甲基吗啡啉	109-02-4	$C_5H_{11}NO$ 101.15	b. p. 115.4	易溶于水
氢氧化钠	NaOH 1310-73-2	NaOH 40.00	m. p. 318.4	易溶于水、乙醇和甘油,不溶于乙醚、丙酮
1-羟基苯并三唑	2592-95-2	$C_6H_5N_3O$ 135.12	m. p. 156~159	可溶于 DMSO(少许)、甲醇(少许)
3-氨基-4-环丁基-2-羟基丁酰胺盐酸盐(化合物 6)	394735-23-0	$C_8H_{17}ClN_2O_2$ 208.69	m. p. 196~200	可溶于 DMSO(少许)、甲醇(少许)
戴斯-马丁氧化剂	87413-09-0	$C_{13}H_{13}IO_8$ 424.14	m. p. 130~133	微溶于 CH_2Cl_2、$CHCl_3$、MeCN 和 THF
波普瑞韦(化合物 1)	394730-60-0	$C_{27}H_{45}N_5O_5$ 519.68	m. p. 107(分解)	DMSO:16.67~100 mg/mL H_2O:< 0.1 mg/mL 乙醇:~100 mg/mL

2. 合成路线

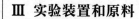

波普瑞韦（化合物 **1**）的合成以叔亮氨酸脲（化合物 **2**）、二甲基环丙基脯氨酸类似物（化合物 **3**）为原料，以 EDC·HCl 为缩合剂，经酰胺化反应获得中间体化合物 **4**，该中间体水解后得到化合物 **5**。随后，所获得的化合物 **5** 再与外消旋的 β-氨基酰胺（化合物 **6**）发生酰胺化反应获得化合物 **7**，最后，用戴斯-马丁氧化剂处理化合物 **7** 后获得目标化合物 **1**。

安全提示： 戴斯-马丁氧化剂（DMP）在撞击或加热到 ＞130 ℃ 时可能会爆炸，所有与 DMP 相关的操作需在冷却条件下完成。

3. 知识点

酰化反应，水解反应，氧化反应，EDC·HCl，戴斯-马丁氧化剂。

酰化装置

Ⅲ 实验装置和原料

1. 实验装置

酰化装置由磁力搅拌器、冰水浴、三口烧瓶、回流冷凝管和温度计组成。

2. 原料

合成产物	原料			
	名称	用量	试剂级别	用途
化合物 4	(S)-2-(3-(叔丁基)脲基)-3,3-二甲基丁酸	10.08 g(0.0438 mol)	—	反应物
	(1R,2S,5S)-6,6-二甲基-3-氮杂双环[3.1.0]己烷-2-羧酸甲酯盐酸盐	9 g(0.0438 mol)	—	反应物
	N,N-二甲基甲酰胺	45 mL	分析纯	溶剂
	甲苯	45 mL	分析纯	溶剂
	1-乙基-3-(3-二甲基氨基丙基)碳酰二亚胺盐酸盐（EDC·HCl）	10.89 g(0.0567 mol)	分析纯	反应物
	N-甲基吗啡啉	11.07 g(0.1092 mol)	分析纯	碱
	蒸馏水	135 mL	—	溶剂
	1 mol/L 盐酸溶液	45 mL	自制	调 pH 值
	10%碳酸氢钠溶液	45 mL	自制	调 pH 值

合成产物	原料			
	名称	用量	试剂级别	用途
化合物 5	化合物 4	5 g(0.0131 mol)	—	反应物
	甲苯	50 mL	分析纯	溶剂
	甲醇	5 mL	分析纯	溶剂
	47％氢氧化钠溶液	1.58 mL	自制	碱
	蒸馏水	25 mL	—	溶剂
	1 mol/L 盐酸溶液	25 mL	自制	调 pH 值
	乙酸乙酯	50 mL	分析纯	溶剂
	甲基叔丁基醚	25 mL	分析纯	溶剂
化合物 7	化合物 5	4 g(0.0108 mol)	—	反应物
	3-氨基-4-环丁基-2-羟基丁酰胺盐酸盐	2.5 g(0.0119 mol)	—	反应物
	乙酸乙酯	32 mL	分析纯	溶剂
	N,N-二甲基甲酰胺	8 mL	分析纯	溶剂
	1-乙基-3-(3-二甲基氨基丙基)碳酰二亚胺盐酸盐	2.5 g(0.013 mol)	分析纯	反应物
	1-羟基苯并三唑	0.3 g(0.0022 mol)	分析纯	外消旋化抑制剂
	N-甲基吗啉	2.75 g(0.0271 mol)	分析纯	碱
	蒸馏水	30 mL		溶剂
	1 mol/L 盐酸溶液	20 mL	自制	调 pH 值
	10％ NaHCO$_3$ 溶液	20 mL	自制	调 pH 值
	正庚烷	24 mL	分析纯	溶剂
波普瑞韦 (化合物 1)	化合物 7	2 g(0.0038 mol)	—	反应物
	乙酸乙酯	35 mL	分析纯	溶剂
	戴斯-马丁氧化剂	2.6 g(0.0061 mol)	分析纯	氧化剂
	甲基叔丁基醚	10 mL	分析纯	溶剂
	40％亚硫酸氢钠溶液	适量		抗氧剂
	庚烷	24 mL	分析纯	溶剂

Ⅳ 实验操作

1. 化合物 4 的制备

（1）搭建酰化装置。

（2）将干燥的 100 mL 三口烧瓶置于冰水浴中，0~10 ℃下保持搅拌，加入 10.08 g(S)-2-(3-(叔丁基) 脲基)-3,3-二甲基丁酸、9 g(1R，2S，5S)-6,6-二甲基-3-氮杂双环［3.1.0］己烷-2-羧酸甲酯盐酸盐、90 mL DMF-甲苯混合溶液（体积比 1：1）。然后，加入 10.89 g EDC·HCl 和 11.07 g N-甲基吗啉。

（3）将反应混合物在 0~10 ℃下搅拌 4~5 h。

（4）反应完成后，在 0~10 ℃ 下缓慢加入 90 mL 水。分出有机层，有机层用 45 mL 1 mol/L HCl 溶液、45 mL 10％ NaHCO$_3$ 溶液、45 mL 水和 45 mL 盐水依次洗涤。随后用无水硫酸钠干燥。

（5）过滤，旋转蒸发除去溶剂，得到白色固体，干燥，称重。

2. 化合物 5 的制备

（1）搭建酰化装置。

（2）将干燥的 100 mL 三口烧瓶置于冰水浴中，0～10 ℃下保持搅拌，加入 50 mL 甲苯、5 g 化合物 **4**、5 mL 甲醇和 1.58 mL 47%氢氧化钠溶液。

（3）加完后，将温度缓慢升至 25～30 ℃，并将反应物在该温度下搅拌 3～4 h。

（4）反应完成后，向反应混合物中加入 25 mL 水，并分离水层。

（5）用 25 mL 1 mol/L HCl 溶液将水层酸化至 pH＝2，并用乙酸乙酯（2×25 mL）萃取产物。干燥。

（6）将有机层减压蒸发浓缩至 80%，并于 5～10 ℃下加入预冷的 25 mL 甲基叔丁基醚。

（7）将物料在 5～10 ℃下搅拌 2～3 h。

（8）过滤，得到白色固体，干燥，称重。

3. 化合物 7 的制备

（1）搭建酰化装置。

（2）将干燥的 100 mL 三口烧瓶置于冰水浴中，0～10 ℃下保持搅拌，加入 4 g 化合物 **5**，2.5 g 3-氨基-4-环丁基-2-羟基丁酰胺盐酸盐（化合物 **6**）、32 mL 乙酸乙酯和 8 mL DMF，搅拌溶解。然后，加入 2.5 g EDC·HCl、0.3 g 1-羟基苯并三唑和 2.75 g N-甲基吗啉。

（3）将反应混合物在 0～10 ℃下搅拌 5～6 h。

（4）反应完成后，在 0～10 ℃下加入 30 mL 水。分出有机层，有机层用 20 mL 1 mol/L HCl 溶液洗涤，然后用 20 mL 10% NaHCO$_3$溶液洗涤。分出有机层，干燥。

（5）将有机层减压蒸发浓缩至 80%，并于 0～10 ℃下加入预冷的 24 mL 庚烷。

（6）过滤，得到白色至灰白色固体，干燥，称重。

4. 波普瑞韦（化合物 1）的制备

（1）搭建酰化装置。

（2）将干燥的 100 mL 三口烧瓶置于冰水浴中，0～10 ℃下保持搅拌，加入 2 g 化合物 **7**、20 mL 乙酸乙酯。然后，分三批以 45 min 的相等间隔添加 2.6 g 戴斯-马丁氧化剂。

（3）将反应混合物在 12～18 ℃下搅拌 3 h。

（4）反应完成后，将反应物在真空下通过硅藻土过滤。用水洗涤滤液，并将 40%的亚硫酸氢钠溶液添加到有机层中。

（5）将溶液在 25～30 ℃下搅拌 12～15 h。分出有机层，干燥。

（6）将有机层减压蒸发浓缩至 80%，加入 8 mL 环己烷。在 25～30 ℃下搅拌混合物 1 h。

（7）过滤，得到亚硫酸盐加合物。

（8）将亚硫酸盐加合物溶解在 5 mL 水 和 10 mL 乙酸乙酯的混合溶剂中，并冷却至 0～3 ℃，搅拌 10～15 min。

（9）分离出水层。在 0～3 ℃下用 5 mL 乙酸乙酯洗涤水层。在水层中加入

10 mL甲基叔丁基醚，并在25～30 ℃下搅拌反应物质2～3 h。分出有机层，干燥。

（10）将有机层减压蒸发浓缩至80％，于0～5 ℃下加入预冷的24 mL庚烷，并在该温度下搅拌30～45 min。

（11）过滤，得到白色固体，干燥，称重，计算收率，测熔点。

（12）将产物送到指导教师指定的产品回收处。

V 实验结果

1. 收率

（1）计算波普瑞韦的理论产量

$$化合物 \textbf{2} ———— 波普瑞韦$$
$$M_w = 230.30 \text{ g/mol} ———— M_w = 519.68 \text{ g/mol}$$
$$0.0438 \text{ mol} ———— 0.0438 \text{ mol}$$
$$理论产量 = 0.0438 \text{ mol} \times 519.68 \text{ g/mol} = 22.76 \text{ g}$$

（2）计算波普瑞韦的收率

$$收率 = \frac{产品实际产量}{产品理论产量} \times 100\% = \frac{(\quad\quad)}{22.76 \text{ g}} \times 100\% = (\quad\quad)\%$$

2. 产品外观与熔点

A. 外观：_____；

B. 熔点：

理论值：107 ℃（分解）；

实测值：_____。

3. 实验结果分析

_____

_____

_____

_____

_____

_____

_____。

VI 注意事项

1. 为了避免副产物的生成，反应要缓慢升温。

2. 所有实验操作应按照规范操作。

3. 整个反应是接着上一步反应进行的，所用试剂的量需要按照比例计算后使用。

VII 产物的含量测定

色谱条件：Poroshell色谱柱，100 mm×4.6 mm，柱粒径2.7 μm；以0.01 mol/L磷酸二氢钠水溶液为缓冲液（用氢氧化钠溶液调节pH值为7.0）。缓冲液：甲醇为90∶10（体积比）的溶液为流动相A，缓冲液：甲醇为80∶20（体积比）的溶液为流动相 B。梯度为 0 min：70％A，30％B；10 min：40％A，60％B；15 min：25％A，75％B；35 min：10％A，90％B；41 min：70％A，30％B；50 min：70％A，30％B。柱温 40 ℃，检测波长为 220 nm。

测定法：高效液相色谱法。精密称定供试品溶液，注入液相色谱仪，记录色谱图。[Bhalerao DS，et al. Organic Process Research & Development，2015，19 (11)：1559-1567]

Ⅷ 思考题

1. 在该实验中，化合物 **2** 和 **3** 反应的原理是什么？
2. 用结构式表示，偶联试剂 EDC·HCl 还可以用什么代替？

（桑鹏）

Synthesis of Nirmatrelvir

Background

Nirmatrelvir is a covalent inhibitor of the major protease (Mpro) of severe acute respiratory syndrome coronavirus 2 (SARS-CoV-2). Its combination with Ritonavir is the antiviral drug Paxlovid, which is used clinically for the treatment of mild to moderate coronavirus pneumonia (COVID-19). The chemical structure of Nirmatrelvir is shown in Fig. 16-1.

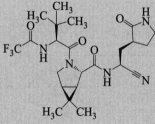

Fig. 16-1 Chemical structure of Nirmatrelvir

The mechanism of action of Nirmatrelvir

I Purposes and Requirements

1. To master the principle of Ugi-type three-component reaction (U-3CR).

2. To master the reaction operations of the Ugi-type three-component reaction, hydrolysis reaction, and cyanation reaction.

3. To understand the mode of action of Nirmatrelvir and its target.

II Principle of the Reaction

1. Physical data of the main reactants and product

Name	Structure CAS No.	Formula M. Wt	b. p. or m. p. / ℃	Solubility
Nirmatrelvir (Compound **1**)	2628280-40-8	$C_{23}H_{32}F_3N_5O_4$ 499.53	m. p. 138~145	The solubility in DMSO is 140 mg/mL, soluble in commonly used organic solvents

Name	Structure CAS No.	Formula M. Wt	b. p. or m. p. / ℃	Solubility
(3S)-3-[(2S)3-(Benzoic acid group)2-Isonitrile propyl]2-pyrrolidone (Compound **2**)	2803923-54-6	$C_{15}H_{16}N_2O_3$ 272. 30	—	Soluble in commonly used organic solvents
3-methyl-*N*-(trifluoroacetyl)-L-valine(Compound **3**)	666832-71-9	$C_8H_{12}F_3NO_3$ 227. 18	m. p. 68～70	Soluble in commonly used organic solvents
(1*R*,5*S*)-6,6-dimethyl-3-azabicyclo [3. 1. 0]hex-2-ene (Compound **4**)	1037559-71-9	$C_7H_{11}N$ 109. 17	b. p. 154.1±13.0	Soluble in commonly used organic solvents
Compound **5**	2803923-55-7	$C_{30}H_{39}F_3N_4O_6$ 608. 65	—	Soluble in commonly used organic solvents
Compound **6**	2803923-56-8	$C_{23}H_{35}F_3N_4O_5$ 504. 54	—	Soluble in commonly used organic solvents
2,2,6,6-Tetramethylpiperidine oxide(TEMPO)	2564-83-2	$C_9H_{18}NO$ 156. 25	m. p. 36～38	The solubility in water at 25 ℃ is 0.03 mol/L，soluble in commonly used organic solvents
(Diacetoxyiodo) benzene	3240-34-4	$C_{10}H_{11}IO_4$ 322. 10	m. p. 163～165	Soluble in most organic solvents

2. Synthetic route

The synthesis of Nirmatrelvir(Compound **1**)was carried out using(3S)-3-[(2S)3-(benzoate) 2-isocyanidopropyl] 2-pyrrolidone (Compound **2**), 3-methyl-*N*-(trifluoroacetyl)-L-valine(Compound **3**), and(1R,5S)-6,6-dimethyl-3-azabicyclo[3.1.0]hex-2-ene(Compound **4**)as starting materials. Intermediate compound **5** was obtained through the Ugi-type three-component reaction, followed by hydrolysis to obtain compound **6**, and then the target compound **1** was obtained through a cyanation reaction.

Safety tips: 2,2,6,6-tetramethylpiperidine oxide (TEMPO) has an amine-like odor and can cause serious skin burns and eye damage. When heated rapidly, it forms an explosive mixture with air and may produce harmful gases or vapors when ignited. After inhalation, the injured person should be moved to fresh air, and washed away with plenty of water after eye contact. All operations related to TEMPO must be standardized.

3. Knowledge points

Ugi-type three-component reaction, hydrolysis reaction, cyanation reaction, TEMPO.

Ⅲ Experimental Equipments and Raw Materials

1. Experimental equipment

The Ugi-type three-component reaction apparatus is composed of a magnetic stirrer, a three-necked round-bottom flask, a reflux condenser, and a thermometer.

U-3CR apparatus

2. Raw materials

Synthetic product	Raw materials			
	Name	Quantity	Quality	Use
Compound 5	(3S)-3-[(2S)-3-(Benzoic acid group)-2-Isonitrile propyl]-2-pyrrolidone(Compound **2**)	1.089 g (4 mmol)	AR	Reactant
	3-methyl-*N*-(trifluoroacetyl)-L-valine(Compound **3**)	2 g (8.8 mmol)	AR	Reactant

Synthetic product	Raw materials			
	Name	Quantity	Quality	Use
Compound 5	(1R,5S)-6,6-dimethyl-3-azabicyclo[3.1.0]hex-2-ene(Compound 4)	1.876 g (8.8 mmol)	AR	Solvent
	Dichloromethane	600 mL	CP	Solvent
	Methanol	40 mL	AR	Solvent
	Distilled water	250 mL	—	Solvent
	Saturated sodium bicarbonate solution	250 mL	CP	Neutralizer
	Saturated saline solution	250 mL	CP	For washing
	0.25 mol/L Dilute hydrochloric acid	400 mL	CP	Acid
	0.5 mol/L Sodium hydroxide solution	20 mL	CP	Base
Compound 6	Compound 5	1.556 g (2.556 mmol)	Product prepared	Reactant
	Dichloromethane	400 mL	CP	Solvent
	Methanol	30 mL	AR	Solvent
	Saturated ammonium chloride solution	30 mL	CP	Quenching agent
	Distilled water	30 mL	—	Quenching agent
	Ethyl acetate	250 mL	CP	Extraction solution
	Potassium carbonate	1.237 g (8.951 mmol)	CP	Base
Nirmatrelvir (Compound 1)	Compound 6	897 mg (1.78 mmol)	Product prepared	Reactant
	Dichloromethane	400 mL	CP	Solvent
	Methanol	30 mL	AR	Solvent
	Acetonitrile	16 mL	CP	Solvent
	Distilled water	125 mL	—	For washing
	Saturated saline solution	100 mL	Product prepared	For washing
	Ethyl acetate	120 mL	CP	Solvent
	35%(mass fraction)Sodium thiosulfate	25 mL	CP	Quenching agent
	TEMPO	13.9 mg (0.09 mmol)	CP	Radical Scavenger
	(Diacetoxyiodo)benzene	1.260 g (3.91 mmol)	CP	Oxidizing Agent
	Ammonium acetate	548 mg (7.11 mmol)	CP	Reactant

Ⅳ Operations

1. Preparation of compound 5

(1) Equip the U-3CR apparatus.

(2) In the dry 100 mL three-necked flask, add 1.876 g(1R, 5S)-6,6-dimethyl-3-azabicyclo[3.1.0]hex-2-ene (compound **4**), 20 mL 0.5 mol/L NaOH (aq.), stir at room temperature to dissolve, then add 2 g 3-methyl-N-(trifluoroacetyl)-L-valine (compound **3**), 1.089 g isocyanide (compound **2**), and 8 mL CH_2Cl_2 solution.

(3) Stir the reaction mixture at room temperature for 48 h.

(4) After the reaction is complete, dilute the reaction mixture with 200 mL of CH_2Cl_2 and wash sequentially with 0.25 mol/L HCl (200 mL×2), saturated $NaHCO_3$ aqueous solution (250 mL), water (250 mL), and saturated saline solution (250 mL). Separate the organic layer and dry it over anhydrous sodium sulfate.

(5) Filter, rotary evaporate to remove solvent, and separate by column chromatography to obtain a white solid (eluent: 2% ~ 3% MeOH/CH_2Cl_2), dry, and weigh it.

2. Preparation of compound 6

(1) Equip the U-3CR apparatus.

(2) In the dry 100 mL three-necked flask, add 1.556 g of compound **5** and 51 mL of MeOH, stir to dissolve at room temperature, and then add 1.237 mg of K_2CO_3.

(3) Stir the mixture at room temperature for 1.5 h.

(4) After the reaction is completed, add 30 mL of saturated NH_4Cl solution to the reaction mixture to quench the reaction, and then add 30 mL of water for further dilution.

(5) Extract the aqueous layer with ethyl acetate (50 mL×5), combine the organic layers, and dry over anhydrous Na_2SO_4.

(6) Filter, rotary evaporate to remove solvent, and separate by column chromatography to obtain a white solid (eluent: 5% ~ 7% MeOH/CH_2Cl_2), dry, and weigh it.

3. Preparation of Nirmatrelvir (Compound 1)

(1) Equip the U-3CR apparatus.

(2) In the dry 100 mL three-necked flask, add 897 mg of compound 6 and 18.8 mL of CH_3CN-H_2O (9:1) solution, stir at room temperature to dissolve, then add 13.9 mg of TEMPO, 1.260 g of (diacetoxyiodo) benzene, and 548 mg of NH_4OAc in sequence.

(3) Stir at room temperature for 2 h and detect the end-point of the reaction using TLC (staining with anisaldehyde).

(4) After the reaction is complete, first quench the reaction mixture with 25 mL 35% $Na_2S_2O_3$ solution and then further dilute it with 25 mL water. Extract

the aqueous layer with ethyl acetate （30 mL×4）, combine the organic layers, wash with 100 mL of water and 100 mL of saturated saline solution, separate the organic layer, and dry with Na_2SO_4.

（5）Filter, rotary evaporate to remove solvent, and separate by column chromatography to obtain a white solid （eluent: 2%~4% $MeOH/CH_2Cl_2$）, dry and weigh it, calculate the yield, and measure the melting point.

（6）Send the final product to the place where the teachers designated.

Ⅴ Experimental Results

1. Yield

（1）Calculate the theoretical production of Nirmatrelvir

$$\text{Compound } \mathbf{2} \text{ ———— Nirmatrelvir}$$
$$M_w = 272.30 \text{ g/mol} \text{ ————} M_w = 499.53 \text{ g/mol}$$
$$0.004 \text{ mol} \text{ ————} 0.004 \text{ mol}$$

Theoretical production = 0.004 mol×499.53 g/mol = 2.00 g

（2）Calculate the percent yield of Nirmatrelvir

$$\text{Yield} = \frac{\text{Practical production}}{\text{Theoretical production}} \times 100\% = \frac{(\quad)}{2.00 \text{ g}} \times 100\% = (\quad)\%$$

2. Appearance and melting point of product

A. Appearance: _____ ;

B. m. p. :

Theoretical value: 138~145 ℃ ;

Practical value: _____ .

3. Analysis of experimental results

_____
_____
_____
_____
_____
_____
_____ .

Ⅵ Notes

1. All experimental operations should be carried out in accordance with the specifications.

2. The entire reaction proceeds from the previous step, and the amount of each reagent used needs to be calculated proportionally before use.

Ⅶ Determination of Product Content

Chromatographic conditions: HPLC analysis was performed on an Agilent 1260 series HPLC with a Lux 5u Cellulose-2 column （250 mm×4.6 mm, 5 μm） at a flow rate of 1.25 mL/min using 50% isopropanol/50% hexanes. Spectral data at 210 nm were collected.

Measurement method: Accurately weigh the test sample, inject it into the liquid chromatograph, and record the chromatogram. Calculate the peak area. [Caravez J C, et al. Organic Letters (2022), 24 (49), 9049-9053]

Ⅷ Discussion Questions

1. What is the difference between the Ugi reaction and the U-3CR in this experiment?

2. Is the free radical scavenger TEMP stable? Why?

(By Yan Shi)

实验十六

奈玛特韦的合成

背景知识

奈玛特韦（Nirmatrelvir）是严重急性呼吸综合征冠状病毒 2（SARS-CoV-2）主蛋白酶（Mpro）的共价抑制剂，其与利托那韦（Ritonavir）的复方制剂为抗病毒药物帕罗韦德（Paxlovid），临床用于轻至中度冠状病毒肺炎（COVID-19）的治疗。奈玛特韦的化学结构如图 16-1 所示。

图 16-1　奈玛特韦的化学结构

奈玛特韦的
作用机制

Ⅰ　目的与要求

1. 掌握乌吉三组分反应（Ugi-type three-component reaction，U-3CR）的原理。
2. 掌握乌吉三组分反应、水解反应和氰基化反应的操作。
3. 了解奈玛特韦与靶标的作用方式。

Ⅱ　实验原理

1. 主要反应物和产物的物理常数

名称	结构式 CAS 号	分子式 分子量	沸点或 熔点/℃	溶解性
奈玛特韦（化合物 1）	2628280-40-8	$C_{23}H_{32}F_3N_5O_4$ 499.53	m. p. 138～145	DMSO 中溶解度为 140 mg/mL，易溶于常用有机溶剂

名称	结构式 CAS 号	分子式 分子量	沸点或 熔点/℃	溶解性
(3*S*)-3-[(2*S*)3- (苯甲酸基)2-异腈丙基] 2-吡咯烷酮(化合物 **2**)	2803923-54-6	$C_{15}H_{16}N_2O_3$ 272.30	—	易溶于常用有机溶剂
3-甲基-*N*-(三氟乙酰 基)-L-缬氨酸 (化合物 **3**)	666832-71-9	$C_8H_{12}F_3NO_3$ 227.18	m. p. 68~70	易溶于常用有机溶剂
(1*R*,5*S*)-6,6-二甲基- 3-氮杂双环[3.1.0]己- 2-烯(化合物 **4**)	1037559-71-9	$C_7H_{11}N$ 109.17	b. p. 154.1±13.0	易溶于常用有机溶剂
化合物 **5**	2803923-55-7	$C_{30}H_{39}F_3N_4O_6$ 608.65	—	易溶于常用有机溶剂
化合物 **6**	2803923-56-8	$C_{23}H_{35}F_3N_4O_5$ 504.54	—	易溶于常用有机溶剂
2,2,6,6-四甲基哌啶 氧化物(TEMPO)	2564-83-2	$C_9H_{18}NO$ 156.25	m. p. 36~38	25 ℃水中的溶解度 为 0.03 mol/L,溶于多 种有机溶剂
(二乙酰氧基碘)苯	3240-34-4	$C_{10}H_{11}IO_4$ 322.10	m. p. 163~165	能够溶于大多数有机 溶剂

2. 合成路线

（反应路线图）

奈玛特韦（化合物 **1**）的合成以（3S）-3-[（2S）3-（苯甲酸基）2-异腈丙基]2-吡咯烷酮（化合物 **2**）、3-甲基-N-（三氟乙酰基）-L-缬氨酸（化合物 **3**）和（1R，5S）-6,6-二甲基-3-氮杂双环[3.1.0]己-2-烯（化合物 **4**）为原料，经乌吉三组分反应获得中间体化合物 **5**，然后，经水解得到化合物 **6**，再经氰基化反应获得目标化合物 **1**。

安全提示：2,2,6,6-四甲基哌啶氧化物（TEMPO）有氨样气味，易造成严重皮肤灼伤和眼损伤，在急剧加热下会与空气形成具爆炸性的混合物，起火时可能产生危害性气体或蒸气，吸入之后应将伤者转移到空气新鲜处，眼睛接触之后应用大量清水冲洗。所有与 TEMPO 相关的操作须规范操作。

3. 知识点

乌吉三组分反应，水解反应，氰基化反应，TEMPO。

Ⅲ 实验装置和原料

1. 实验装置

乌吉三组分反应装置由磁力搅拌器、三口烧瓶、回流冷凝管和温度计组成。

2. 原料

乌吉三组分
反应装置

合成产物	原料			
	名称	用量	试剂级别	用途
化合物 **5**	（3S）-3-[（2S）3-（苯甲酸基）2-异腈丙基]2-吡咯烷酮（化合物 **2**）	1.089 g（4 mmol）	分析纯	反应物
	3-甲基-N-（三氟乙酰基）-L-缬氨酸（化合物 **3**）	2 g（8.8 mmol）	分析纯	反应物
	（1R，5S）-6,6-二甲基-3-氮杂双环[3.1.0]己-2-烯（化合物 **4**）	1.876 g（8.8 mmol）	分析纯	反应物
	二氯甲烷	600 mL	化学纯	溶剂
	甲醇	40 mL	分析纯	溶剂

合成产物	原料			
	名称	用量	试剂级别	用途
化合物5	蒸馏水	250 mL	—	溶剂
	饱和碳酸氢钠	250 mL	化学纯	中和试剂
	饱和食盐水	250 mL	化学纯	洗液
	0.25 mol/L 盐酸	400 mL	化学纯	酸
	0.5 mol/L 氢氧化钠	20 mL	化学纯	碱
化合物6	化合物5	1.556 g(2.556 mmol)	自制	反应物
	二氯甲烷	400 mL	化学纯	溶剂
	甲醇	30 mL	分析纯	溶剂
	饱和氯化铵溶液	30 mL	化学纯	淬灭剂
	蒸馏水	30 mL	—	淬灭剂
	乙酸乙酯	250 mL	化学纯	萃取剂
	碳酸钾	1.237 g(8.951 mmol)	化学纯	碱
奈玛特韦(化合物1)	化合物6	897 mg(1.78 mmol)	自制	反应物
	二氯甲烷	400 mL	化学纯	溶剂
	甲醇	30 mL	分析纯	溶剂
	乙腈	16 mL	化学纯	溶剂
	蒸馏水	125 mL	—	洗液
	饱和食盐水	100 mL	自制	洗液
	乙酸乙酯	120 mL	化学纯	溶剂
	35%(质量分数)硫代硫酸钠	25 mL	化学纯	淬灭剂
	TEMPO	13.9 mg(0.09 mmol)	化学纯	自由基捕获剂
	(二乙酰氧基碘)苯	1.260 g(3.91 mmol)	化学纯	氧化剂
	醋酸铵	548 mg(7.11 mmol)	化学纯	反应物

Ⅳ 实验操作

1. 化合物5的制备

（1）搭建乌吉三组分反应装置。

（2）在干燥的100 mL三口烧瓶中，加入1.876 g(1R,5S)-6,6-二甲基-3-氮杂双环[3.1.0]己-2-烯（化合物4）、20 mL 0.5 mol/L NaOH(aq.)，室温搅拌溶解后，加入2 g 3-甲基-N-（三氟乙酰基）-L-缬氨酸（化合物3）、1.089 g异氰化物（化合物2）、8 mL CH₂Cl₂溶液。

（3）将反应混合物在室温条件，搅拌48 h。

（4）反应完成后，加入200 mL CH₂Cl₂稀释反应混合物，依次用0.25 mol/L HCl（200 mL×2）、饱和NaHCO₃水溶液（250 mL）、水（250 mL）和饱和食盐水（250 mL）洗涤。分离有机层，无水硫酸钠干燥。

（5）过滤，旋转蒸发除去溶剂，柱色谱分离得到白色固体（洗脱剂：2%～

3％ MeOH／CH$_2$Cl$_2$），干燥，称重。

2. 化合物 6 的制备

（1）搭建乌吉三组分反应装置。

（2）在干燥的 100 mL 三口烧瓶中，加入 1.556 g 化合物 **5** 和 51 mLMeOH，室温搅拌溶解后，加入 1.237 mg K$_2$CO$_3$。

（3）混合物在室温下搅拌 1.5 h。

（4）反应完成后，向反应混合物中加入 30 mL 饱和 NH$_4$Cl 溶液，淬灭反应，然后加入 30 mL 水进一步稀释。

（5）用乙酸乙酯（50 mL×5）萃取水层，合并有机层，无水 Na$_2$SO$_4$ 干燥。

（6）过滤，旋转蒸发除去溶剂，柱色谱分离得到白色固体（洗脱剂：5％～7％ MeOH／CH$_2$Cl$_2$），干燥，称重。

3. 奈玛特韦（化合物 1）的制备

（1）搭建乌吉三组分反应装置。

（2）在干燥的 100 mL 三口烧瓶中，加入 897 mg 化合物 **6**、18.8 mL CH$_3$CN-H$_2$O（9∶1）的溶液，室温搅拌溶解后，再依次加入 13.9 mg TEMPO、1.260 g（二乙酰氧基碘）苯和 548 mg NH$_4$OAc。

（3）室温搅拌 2 h，用 TLC 检测反应终点（对茴香醛染色）。

（4）反应完成后，先在反应混合物中加入 25 mL 35％的 Na$_2$S$_2$O$_3$ 溶液淬灭反应，再加入 25 mL 水进一步稀释。然后用乙酸乙酯（30 mL×4）萃取，合并有机层，再用 100 mL 水和 100 mL 盐水洗涤，分离有机层，无水硫酸钠干燥。

（5）过滤，旋转蒸发除去溶剂，柱色谱分离得到白色固体（洗脱剂：2％～4％ MeOH／CH$_2$Cl$_2$），干燥，称重，计算收率，测熔点。

（6）将产物送到指导教师指定的产品回收处。

V 实验结果

1. 收率

（1）计算奈玛特韦的理论产量

$$化合物\ \textbf{2} \text{———————} 奈玛特韦$$
$$M_w = 272.30\ g/mol \text{———————} M_w = 499.53\ g/mol$$
$$0.004\ mol \text{———————} 0.004\ mol$$

$$理论产量 = 0.004\ mol × 499.53\ g/mol = 2.00\ g$$

（2）计算奈玛特韦的收率

$$收率 = \frac{产品实际产量}{产品理论产量} × 100\% = \frac{(\quad\quad)}{2.00\ g} × 100\% = (\quad\quad)\%$$

2. 产品外观与熔点

A. 外观：＿＿＿＿＿＿＿＿＿＿＿＿＿＿＿＿＿＿＿＿；

B. 熔点：

　　理论值：138～145 ℃；

　　实测值：＿＿＿＿＿＿＿＿＿＿＿＿＿＿＿＿。

3. 实验结果分析

＿＿＿＿＿＿＿＿＿＿＿＿＿＿＿＿＿＿＿＿＿＿＿＿＿＿＿＿＿＿＿＿＿＿＿＿＿＿＿

＿＿＿＿＿＿＿＿＿＿＿＿＿＿＿＿＿＿＿＿＿＿＿＿＿＿＿＿＿＿＿＿＿＿＿＿＿＿＿

————————————————————————————————————

————————————————————————————————————

————————————————————————————————————

————————————————————————————————————

————————————————————————————————————

——————————————————————————————————。

Ⅵ 注意事项

1. 所有实验操作应按照规范操作进行。

2. 整个反应是接着上一步反应进行的，所用试剂的量需要按照比例计算后使用。

Ⅶ 产物的含量测定

色谱条件：在 Agilent 1260 系列 HPLC 上使用 Lux 5u Cellulose-2 柱（250 mm×4.6 mm，5 μm），以 1.25 mL/min 的流速，使用 50% 异丙醇/50% 己烷进行 HPLC 分析。收集 210 nm 的光谱数据。

测定法：精密称定供试品溶液，注入液相色谱仪，记录色谱图。［Caravez J C，et al. Organic Letters（2022），24（49），9049-9053］

Ⅷ 思考题

1. 试解释乌吉反应和本实验中乌吉三组分反应（U-3CR）的区别。

2. 自由基捕获剂 TEMP 稳定吗？为什么？

（石岩）

Experiment 17

Synthesis of Sofosbuvir

Background

Sofosbuvir is a hepatitis C virus (HCV) RNA polymerase inhibitor. As a prodrug, Sofosbuvir exerts antiviral effects through its *in vivo* metabolite 2′-deoxy-2′-α-fluoride-β-C-methyluridine-5′-monophosphate, and is clinically used for the treatment of chronic hepatitis C. The chemical structure of Sofosbuvir is shown in Fig. 17-1.

The mechanism of action of Sofosbuvir

Fig. 17-1   Chemical structure of Sofosbuvir

Ⅰ Purposes and Requirements

1. To master the reaction principles of glycosylation, debenzoylated protection, and nucleoside phosphoramide prodrug.

2. To master the experimental operations of glycosylation, debenzoylated protection, and nucleoside phosphoramide prodrug.

3. To understand the mode of action of Sofosbuvir and its target.

Ⅱ Principle of the Reaction

1. Physical data of the main reactants and product

Name	Structure CAS No.	Formula M. Wt	b. p. or m. p. /℃	Solubility
Sofosbuvir (Compound **1**)	1190307-88-0	$C_{22}H_{29}FN_3O_9P$ 529.45	m. p. 122~124	Slightly soluble in water, freely soluble in dehydrated ethanol and acetone, and insoluble in heptane

Name	Structure CAS No.	Formula M. Wt	b. p. or m. p. /℃	Solubility
(2R)-2-Deoxy-2-fluoro-2-methyl-α/β-D-erythrofuranosyl chloride-3,5-dibenzoate (Compound 2)	1199809-23-8	$C_{20}H_{18}ClFO_5$ 392.81	b. p. 487.3±45.0 (Predicted)	—
N^4-enzoylcytosine (Compound 3)	26661-13-2	$C_{11}H_9N_3O_2$ 215.21	m. p. >300	Soluble in acidic aqueous solution (slightly heated)
(2R')-N-Benzoyl-2'-deoxy-2'-fluoro-2'-methylcytidine 3',5'-dibenzoate (Compound 4)	817204-32-3	$C_{31}H_{26}FN_3O_7$ 571.55	m. p. 241	Insoluble in water
2'-Deoxy-2'-fluoro-2'-C-methyluridine (Compound 5)	863329-66-2	$C_{10}H_{13}FN_2O_5$ 260.22	m. p. 237~238	Slightly soluble in DMSO and methanol
N-[(S)-(2,3,4,5,6-pentafluorophenoxy)phenoxyphosphoryl]-L-alanine isopropyl ester(Compound 6)	1334513-02-8	$C_{18}H_{17}F_5NO_5P$ 453.08	m. p. 442.6	Soluble in organic solvents such as tetrahydrofuran
Hexamethyldisilazane	999-97-3	$C_6H_{19}NSi_2$ 161.39	b. p. 125	Soluble in organic solvents
Ammonium sulphate	$(NH_4)_2SO_4$ 7783-20-2	$H_8N_2O_4S$ 132.14	m. p. 235~280 (decompose)	Water: 70.6 g/100 mL at 0 ℃, 75.4 g/100 mL at 20 ℃
Stannic chloride	$SnCl_4$ 7646-78-8	$SnCl_4$ 260.513	b. p. 114	Soluble in water

Name	Structure CAS No.	Formula M. Wt	b. p. or m. p. /℃	Solubility
Chlorobenzene	(structure) 108-90-7	C_6H_5Cl 112.56	b. p. 132	Insoluble in water, soluble in most organic solvents
tert-Butylmagnesium chloride(1.7 mol/L)in Tetrahydrofuran	C_4H_9ClMg 677-22-5	C_4H_9ClMg 116.87	m. p. —108	Dissolve with ethanol and water

2. Synthetic route

The synthesis of Sofosbuvir (compound **1**) was carried out using (2R)-2-deoxy-2-fluoro-2-methyl-α/β-D-erythrofuranosyl chloride-3,5-dibenzoate (compound **2**) and N^4-benzoylcytosine (compound **3**) as raw materials. Intermediate compound **4** was obtained through a glycosylation reaction, followed by debenzoylated to obtain compound **5**, which was then phosphorylated with chiral phosphoramidite ester (compound **6**) to obtain the target compound **1**.

Safety Tips: This experiment will come into contact with acetic acid and methanol solutions of ammonia. During operation, attention should be paid to ventilation, strict adherence to operating procedures, and wearing goggles and rubber acid and alkali-resistant gloves. If accidental skin contact occurs, contaminated clothing should be immediately removed and rinsed with running water for 15 minutes. If there are burns, seek medical treatment. When in contact with the eyes, immediately lift the eyelids and rinse with flowing water or saline solution for at least 15 minutes before seeking medical attention.

3. Knowledge points

Glycosylation reaction, debenzoylated protection reaction, phosphorylation reaction, nucleoside prodrug technology.

Ⅲ Experimental Equipments and Raw Materials

1. Experimental equipment

The glycosylation reaction apparatus is composed of a magnetic stirrer, a three-necked round-bottom flask, a reflux condenser, and a thermometer.

The phosphorylation reaction apparatus is composed of a magnetic stirrer, an ice-water bath, a three-necked round-bottom flask, a reflux condenser, and a thermometer.

The glycosylation reaction apparatus and the phosphsorylation reaction apparatus

2. Raw materials

Synthetic product	Raw materials			
	Name	Quantity	Quality	Use
Compound 4	(2R)-2-Deoxy-2-fluoro-2-methyl-α/β-D-erythrofuranosyl chloride-3,5-dibenzoate (Compound 2)	18 g (0.046 mol)	CP	Reactant
	N^4-enzoylcytosine (Compound 3)	11.87 g (0.055 mol)	CP	Reactant
	Hexamethyldisilazane	8.87 g (0.055 mol)	CP	Solvent
	Ammonium sulfate	100 mg (0.0008 mol)	CP	Catalyst
	Chlorobenzene	115 mL	CP	Solvent
	Stannic chloride	36 g (0.138 mol)	CP	Catalyst
	Dichloromethane	245 mL	CP	Solvent
	$NaHCO_3$	6.3 g	CP	Base
	Isopropanol	15 mL	CP	Solvent
Compound 5	Compound 4	15 g (0.026 mol)	Product prepared	Reactant
	Acetic acid	150 mL	CP	Reactant
	Saturated methanol solution of ammonia	30 mL	—	Reactant
	Ethyl acetate	25 mL	CP	Solvent
Sofosbuvir (Compound 1)	Compound 5	4.8 g (0.018 mol)	Product prepared	Reactant
	N-[(S)-(2,3,4,5,6-pentafluorophenoxy)phenoxyphosphoryl]-L-alanine isopropyl ester (Compound 6)	10 g (0.022 mol)	CP	Reactant
	tert-Butylmagnesium chloride (1.7 mol/L) in Tetrahydrofuran	22 mL (0.038 mol)	CP	Base
	Tetrahydrofuran	20 mL	CP	Solvent
	1 mol/L HCl	25 mL	Product prepared	Quenching agent
	Toluene	90 mL	CP	Solvent
	Dichloromethane	30 mL	CP	Solvent

Ⅳ Operations

1. Preparation of compound 4

(1) Equip the glycosylation reaction apparatus.

(2) In the dry 250 mL three-necked flask, add 11.87 g of N^4-benzoylcytosine (compound **3**), 100 mg of ammonium sulfate, and 8.87 g of hexamethyldisilazane, and 100 mL of chlorobenzene in sequence while stirring. Heat to 135 ℃ and reflux for 1 h.

(3) Cool to room temperature to obtain O-trimethylsilyl-N^4-benzoylcytosine liquid.

(4) Add 18 g of compound **2** and 36 g of stannic chloride, keep stirring, Heat to 80 ℃ and react for 6 h.

(5) Cool to room temperature, add 100 mL of dichloromethane, and stir evenly. Add the solution to a suspension of 100 mL dichloromethane containing 6.3 g of $NaHCO_3$ solid and 14 g of diatomaceous earth, and stir evenly.

(6) Cool the obtained slurry to 10~15 ℃ and slowly add 16 mL of water to quench the reaction. Slowly raise the temperature to 45 ℃ and heat for 30 min (During the heating process, HCl gas overflows, so needs to be slowly heated).

(7) Cool the slurry to about 15 ℃, filter, and wash the filter cake three times with 10 mL of dichloromethane.

(8) Remove solvent by rotary evaporation.

(9) Add 15 mL of chlorobenzene and 15 mL dichloromethane to the residue, heat to 90 ℃, then slowly cool to about −5 ℃ and let it stand for 2 h.

(10) Filter, wash three times with 5 mL of isopropanol, dry the filter cake in a vacuum oven at 70 ℃ for 5 h to obtain a white solid, and weigh it.

2. Preparation of compound 5

(1) Equip the glycosylation reaction apparatus.

(2) In the dry 250 mL three-necked flask, add 15 g of compound **4** and 150 mL of 70% acetic acid aqueous solution, heat and reflux for 6 h.

(3) Cool to room temperature, add 9 mL of water, stir for 2 h, and precipitate the solid. Filter.

(4) Add the obtained solid into a 100 mL reaction flask, add 30 mL of saturated ammonia methanol solution. Seal the reaction flask and stir at room temperature for 8 h.

(5) Filter the reaction mixture through diatomite and remove the solvent by rotary evaporation to obtain a white solid.

(6) Add the obtained solid into a 100 mL reaction flask, add 15 mL of ethyl acetate, and stir at room temperature for 3 h.

(7) Filter, wash the filter cake with 10 mL of ethyl acetate, dry, and weigh it.

3. Preparation of Sofosbuvir (Compound 1)

(1) Equip the phosphorylation reaction apparatus.

(2) In the dry 100 mL three-necked flask in an ice-water bath, add 4.8 g of compound **5** and 10 mL of tetrahydrofuran, stir and dissolve. Add 22 mL of 1.7 mol/L tert-butyl magnesium chloride in tetrahydrofuran and stir for 30 min. Subsequently, remove the ice-water bath and stir at room temperature for 30 min.

(3) In an ice-water bath, add 10 g of compound **6** and stir at room temperature for 4 h. Then cool the reaction solution to 5 ℃ and add 25 mL 1 mol/L hydrochloric acid to quench the reaction.

(4) Separate the organic layer and extract the aqueous layer with toluene (30 mL×3). Combine the organic layer and dry over anhydrous sodium sulfate.

(5) Filter and evaporate the filtrate by rotary evaporation to about 20 mL. Add 20 mL of dichloromethane to the residue and stir at room temperature for 4 h.

(6) Filter, wash the filter cake with 10 mL of cold dichloromethane (0 ℃) to obtain a white solid, dry, weigh, calculate the yield, and measure the melting point.

(7) Send the final product to the place where the teachers designated.

V Experimental Results

1. Yield

(1) Calculate the theoretical production of Sofosbuvir

$$\text{Compound } \mathbf{2} \text{ ——— Sofosbuvir}$$
$$M_w = 392.81 \text{ g/mol ———} M_w = 529.45 \text{ g/mol}$$
$$0.046 \text{ mol ———} 0.046 \text{ mol}$$

Theoretical production $= 0.046 \text{ mol} \times 529.45 \text{ g/mol} = 24.35 \text{ g}$

(2) Calculate the percent yield of Sofosbuvir

$$\text{Yield} = \frac{\text{Practical production}}{\text{Theoretical production}} \times 100\% = \frac{(\quad)}{24.35 \text{ g}} \times 100\% = (\quad)\%$$

2. Appearance and melting point of product

A. Appearance: _____ ;

B. m. p. :

Theoretical value: 122~124 ℃;

Practical value: _____ .

3. Analysis of experimental results

_____

_____

_____

_____

_____

_____

_____

_____

_____

Ⅵ Notes

1. During the glycosylation process, inorganic salts and isomers of the target product may be generated, which increases the difficulty of removing impurities. Therefore, appropriate post-treatment measures such as acid neutralization, separation and purification need to be taken during the synthesis process to reduce the generation of impurities and isomers and improve the purity of the product.

2. In the synthesis process of Sofosbuvir prodrug, reaction selectivity is a key factor, and high temperature can lead to a decrease in selectivity. Therefore, tert-butyl magnesium chloride was added to an ice-water bath.

3. The entire reaction proceeds from the previous step, and the amount of each reagent used needs to be calculated proportionally before use.

Ⅶ Determination of Product Content

Chromatographic conditions: Using a column (150 mm × 4.6 mm) packed with end-capped, base-deactivated particles of silica gel, the surface of which has been modified with chemically bonded octadecylsilyl groups (3.5 μm). The mobile phase is a mixture of 65% mobile phase A (a mixture of 21 volumes of 0.05% phosphoric acid, 77 volumes of water, and 2 volumes of acetonitrile) and 35% mobile phase B (a mixture of 21 volumes of 0.05% phosphoric acid and 79 volumes of acetonitrile). The flow rate is 1.5 mL/min. The injection volume is 20 μL.

Measurement method: High-performance liquid chromatography method. Accurately weigh 50 mg of the test sample and standard sample, dilute them to 100 mL, and prepare the test sample and standard solution. Inject the test solution and standard solution into the liquid chromatograph and record the chromatogram within 20 min. The retention time of Sofosbuvir is 11 min, and the percentage content is calculated using the external standard method. (《International Pharmacopoeia》11th edition)

Ⅷ Discussion Questions

1. In terms of structure, why does the quenching process of the glycosylation reaction produce gas?

2. Which reagents can replace aminomethanol when removing benzoyl groups in nucleoside drug synthesis?

(By Yonggang Meng)

实验十七

索磷布韦的合成

背景知识

索磷布韦（Sofosbuvir）为丙型肝炎病毒（HCV）RNA 聚合酶抑制剂，作为一种前药，索磷布韦通过其体内代谢物 2′-脱氧-2′-α-氟-β-C-甲基尿苷-5′-单磷酸酯产生抗病毒作用，临床用于慢性丙型肝炎的治疗。索磷布韦的化学结构如图 17-1 所示。

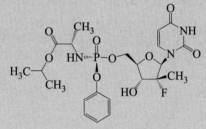

图 17-1　索磷布韦的化学结构

索磷布韦的
作用机制

Ⅰ　目的与要求

1. 掌握糖苷化、脱苯甲酰基保护、核苷-磷酰胺酯前药的反应原理。
2. 掌握糖苷化、脱苯甲酰基保护、核苷-磷酰胺酯前药的实验操作。
3. 了解索磷布韦与靶标的作用方式。

Ⅱ　实验原理

1. 主要反应物和产物的物理常数

名称	结构式 CAS 号	分子式 分子量	沸点或 熔点/℃	溶解性
索磷布韦（化合物 1）	 1190307-88-0	$C_{22}H_{29}FN_3O_9P$ 529.45	m.p. 122~124	微溶于水,易溶于无水乙醇和丙酮,不溶于庚烷

名称	结构式 CAS 号	分子式 分子量	沸点或 熔点/℃	溶解性
(2R)-2-脱氧-2-氟-2-甲基—α/β-D-赤-呋喃戊糖基氯化物-3,5-二苯甲酸酯(化合物2)	1199809-23-8	$C_{20}H_{18}ClFO_5$ 392.81	b. p. 487.3±45.0 (预测)	—
N^4-苯甲酰胞嘧啶 (化合物3)	26661-13-2	$C_{11}H_9N_3O_2$ 215.21	m. p. >300	可溶于酸性水溶液(略微加热)
(2'R)-N-苯甲酰基-2'-脱氧-2'-氟-2'-甲基胞苷 3',5'-二苯甲酸酯 (化合物4)	817204-32-3	$C_{31}H_{26}FN_3O_7$ 571.55	m. p. 241	不溶于水
2'-脱氧-2'-氟-2'-C-甲基尿苷(化合物5)	863329-66-2	$C_{10}H_{13}FN_2O_5$ 260.22	m. p. 237~238	微溶于 DMSO 和甲醇
N-[(S)-(2,3,4,5,6-五氟苯氧基)苯氧基磷酰基]-L-丙氨酸异丙酯 (化合物6)	1334513-02-8	$C_{18}H_{17}F_5NO_5P$ 453.08	m. p. 442.6	溶于四氢呋喃等有机溶剂
六甲基二硅氮烷	999-97-3	$C_6H_{19}NSi_2$ 161.39	b. p. 125	溶于有机溶剂
硫酸铵	$(NH_4)_2SO_4$ 7783-20-2	$H_8N_2O_4S$ 132.14	m. p. 235~280 (分解)	水:0 ℃溶解 70.6 g/100 mL; 20 ℃溶解 75.4 g/100 mL
氯化锡	$SnCl_4$ 7646-78-8	$SnCl_4$ 260.513	b. p. 114	溶于水
氯苯	108-90-7	C_6H_5Cl 112.56	b. p. 132	不溶于水,溶于多数有机溶剂
1.7 mol/L 叔丁基氯化镁的四氢呋喃溶液	C_4H_9ClMg 677-22-5	C_4H_9ClMg 116.87	m. p. -108	与乙醇和水互溶

2. 合成路线

索磷布韦（化合物 **1**）的合成以（2*R*)-2-脱氧-2-氟-2-甲基-α/β-D-赤-呋喃戊糖基氯化物-3,5-二苯甲酸酯（化合物 **2**）和 N^4-苯甲酰胞嘧啶（化合物 **3**）为原料，经糖苷化反应获得中间体化合物 **4**，然后，经脱苯甲酰基得到化合物 **5**，再与手性磷酰胺酯（化合物 **6**）发生磷酸酯化反应得到目标物化合物 **1**。

安全提示：本实验中会接触到冰醋酸、氨的甲醇溶液，在操作中应注意通风，严格遵守操作规程，佩戴护目镜和橡胶耐酸碱手套。如果不小心皮肤接触，应立即脱去污染的衣着，用流动清水冲洗 15 min。若有灼伤，就医治疗。如果眼睛接触，立即提起眼睑，用流动清水或生理盐水冲洗至少 15 min，并就医治疗。

3. 知识点
糖苷化反应，脱苯甲酰基保护反应，磷酸酯化反应，核苷前药技术。

Ⅲ 实验装置和原料

1. 实验装置
糖苷化反应装置由磁力搅拌器、三口烧瓶、回流冷凝管和温度计组成。
磷酸酯化反应装置由磁力搅拌器、冰水浴、三口烧瓶、回流冷凝管和温度计组成。

糖苷化反应装置和磷酸酯化反应装置

2. 原料

合成产物	原料			
	名称	用量	试剂级别	用途
化合物 **4**	（2*R*)-2-脱氧-2-氟-2-甲基-α/β-D-赤-呋喃戊糖基氯化物-3,5-二苯甲酸酯（化合物 **2**）	18 g(0.046 mol)	化学纯	反应物
	N^4-苯甲酰胞嘧啶（化合物 **3**）	11.87 g(0.055 mol)	化学纯	反应物
	六甲基二硅氮烷	8.87 g(0.055 mol)	化学纯	反应物
	硫酸铵	100 mg(0.0008 mol)	化学纯	催化剂
	氯苯	115 mL	化学纯	溶剂

合成产物	原料			
	名称	用量	试剂级别	用途
化合物 4	氯化锡	36 g(0.138 mol)	化学纯	催化剂
	二氯甲烷	245 mL	化学纯	溶剂
	NaHCO$_3$	6.3 g	化学纯	碱
	异丙醇	15 mL	化学纯	溶剂
化合物 5	化合物 4	15 g(0.026 mol)	自制	反应物
	乙酸	150 mL	化学纯	反应物
	氨的甲醇饱和溶液	30 mL	—	反应物
	乙酸乙酯	25 mL	化学纯	溶剂
索磷布韦(化合物 1)	化合物 5	4.8 g(0.018 mol)	自制	反应物
	N-[(S)-(2,3,4,5,6-五氟苯氧基)苯氧基磷酰基]-L-丙氨酸异丙酯(化合物 6)	10 g(0.022 mol)	化学纯	反应物
	1.7 mol/L 叔丁基氯化镁的四氢呋喃溶液	22 mL(0.038 mol)	化学纯	碱
	四氢呋喃	20 mL	化学纯	溶剂
	1 mol/L HCl	25 mL	自制	淬灭剂
	甲苯	90 mL	化学纯	溶剂
	二氯甲烷	30 mL	化学纯	溶剂

Ⅳ 实验操作

1. 化合物 4 的制备

（1）搭建糖苷化反应装置。

（2）在 250 mL 三口烧瓶中，搅拌状态下，依次加入 11.87 g N^4-苯甲酰胞嘧啶（化合物 3）、100 mg 硫酸铵、8.87 g 六甲基二硅氮烷和 100 mL 氯苯，升温至 135 ℃，回流 1 h。

（3）冷却至室温，获得 O-三甲基甲硅烷基-N^4-苯甲酰胞嘧啶液体。

（4）向获得的液体中加入 18 g 化合物 2 和 36 g 氯化锡，保持搅拌，升温至 80 ℃，反应 6 h。

（5）冷却至室温，加入 100 mL 二氯甲烷，搅拌均匀。将该溶液加入含有 6.3 g 碳酸氢钠固体和 14 g 硅藻土的 100 mL 二氯甲烷的悬浮液中，搅拌均匀。

（6）将所得浆液冷却至 10～15 ℃，缓慢加入 16 mL 水淬灭反应。缓慢升温至 45 ℃，加热 30 min（升温过程中，有 HCl 气体溢出，需缓慢加热）。

（7）将浆液冷却至约 15 ℃，过滤，滤饼用 10 mL 二氯甲烷洗涤三次。

（8）旋转蒸发除去溶剂。

（9）残留物中加入 15 mL 氯苯和 15 mL 二氯甲烷，升温至 90 ℃，然后缓慢冷却至约 −5 ℃，静置 2 h。

（10）抽滤，用 5 mL 异丙醇洗涤三次，滤饼置于 70 ℃的真空烘箱内干燥 5 h，得到白色固体，称重。

2. 化合物 5 的制备

(1) 搭建糖苷化反应装置。

(2) 在干燥的 250 mL 三口烧瓶中，加入 15 g 化合物 **4** 和 150 mL 70％乙酸水溶液，加热回流反应 6 h。

(3) 冷却至室温，加入 9 mL 水，搅拌 2 h，析出固体。过滤。

(4) 将所得固体加入 100 mL 反应瓶中，再加入 30 mL 氨-甲醇饱和溶液。密封反应瓶，并在室温下搅拌 8 h。

(5) 将反应混合物通过硅藻土过滤，旋转蒸发除去溶剂，得到白色固体。

(6) 将所得到的固体加入 100 mL 反应瓶中，加入 15 mL 乙酸乙酯，室温搅拌 3 h。

(7) 过滤，用 10 mL 乙酸乙酯洗涤滤饼，干燥，称重。

3. 索磷布韦（化合物 1）的制备

(1) 搭建磷酸酯化反应装置。

(2) 将干燥的 100 mL 三口烧瓶置于冰水浴中，加入 4.8 g 化合物 **5** 和 20 mL 四氢呋喃，搅拌溶解。加入 22 mL 1.7 mol/L 叔丁基氯化镁的四氢呋喃溶液，搅拌 30 min。随后，撤去冰水浴，室温搅拌 30 min。

(3) 冰水浴下，加入 10 g 化合物 **6**，室温搅拌 4 h。然后将反应液冷却至 5 ℃，加入 25 mL 1 mol/L 的盐酸淬灭反应。

(4) 分离有机层，水层用甲苯（30 mL×3）萃取。合并有机相，无水硫酸钠干燥。

(5) 过滤，滤液旋转蒸发至约 20 mL。向残留物中加入 20 mL 二氯甲烷，室温搅拌 4 h。

(6) 过滤，用 10 mL 冷二氯甲烷（0 ℃）洗涤滤饼，得到白色固体，干燥，称重，计算收率，测熔点。

(7) 将产物送到指导教师指定的产品回收处。

V 实验结果

1. 收率

(1) 计算索磷布韦的理论产量。

$$化合物 \textbf{2} \longrightarrow 索磷布韦$$
$$M_w = 392.81 \text{ g/mol} \longrightarrow M_w = 529.45 \text{ g/mol}$$
$$0.046 \text{ mol} \longrightarrow 0.046 \text{ mol}$$

理论产量 = 0.046 mol × 529.45 g/mol = 24.35 g

(2) 计算索磷布韦的收率

$$收率 = \frac{产品实际产量}{产品理论产量} \times 100\% = \frac{(\qquad)}{24.35 \text{ g}} \times 100\% = (\qquad)\%$$

2. 产品外观与熔点

A. 外观：_____；

B. 熔点：

理论值：122～124 ℃；

实测值：_____。

3. 实验结果分析

_____

_____

_____

_____

_____

_____

_____

_____ 。

Ⅵ 注意事项

1. 糖苷化过程中可能会生成无机盐和目标产物的异构体，这增加了去除杂质的难度。因此，在合成过程中需要采取适当的后处理措施，如酸中和、分离纯化等，以减少杂质和异构体的生成，提高产品的纯度。

2. 索磷布韦前药合成过程中，反应选择性是关键因素，温度过高会导致选择性降低，因此选择在冰水浴下加入叔丁基氯化镁。

3. 整个反应是接着上一步反应进行的，所用试剂的量需要按照比例计算后使用。

Ⅶ 产物的含量测定

色谱条件：使用填充有封端的、碱失活硅胶颗粒的改性化学键合十八烷基甲硅烷基（3.5 μm）柱（150 mm×4.6 mm）；流动相为 65% 流动相 A（21 倍体积的 0.05% 磷酸、77 倍体积的水和 2 倍体积的乙腈的混合物）和 35% 流动相 B（21 倍体积的 0.05% 磷酸和 79 倍体积的乙腈的混合物）的混合液；流速为 1.5 mL/min；进样量为 20 μL。

测定法：高效液相色谱法。精密称定 50 mg 供试品和标准品，分别稀释至 100 mL，配置成供试品和标准品溶液。将供试品溶液和标准品溶液，注入液相色谱仪，记录 20 min 内的色谱图，索磷布韦的保留时间为 11 min，采用外标法进行百分含量计算。（《国际药典（第十一版）》）

Ⅷ 思考题

1. 用结构式表示，在淬灭糖苷化反应的过程中，为什么有气体生成？
2. 在核苷药物合成中，脱去苯甲酰基时，哪些试剂可替代氨甲醇？

（孟勇刚）

Experiment 18

Synthesis of Azvudine

Background

Azvudine（FNC）is a viral reverse transcriptase inhibitor. It is a nucleoside antiviral drug with independent intellectual property rights in China. It can be administered orally and used clinically for the treatment of AIDS and COVID-19 infection. The chemical structure of Azvudine is shown in Fig. 18-1.

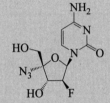

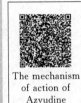

The mechanism of action of Azvudine

Fig. 18-1　Chemical structure of Azvudine

Ⅰ　Purposes and Requirements

1. To master the principle of condensation reaction, ammonolysis reaction, and debenzoylation reaction.

2. To master the experimental operation of the condensation reaction, ammonolysis reaction, and debenzoylation reaction.

3. To understand the mode of action of Azvudine and its target.

Ⅱ　Principle of the Reaction

1. Physical data of the main reactants and product

Name	Structure CAS No.	Formula M. Wt	b. p. or m. p. / ℃	Solubility
Azvudine(Compound **1**)	1011529-10-4	$C_9H_{11}FN_6O_4$ 286. 22	m. p. 99～100	DMSO: 57 ~ 125 mg/mL; water: ~ 57 mg/mL; ethanol: ~57 mg/mL

Name	Structure CAS No.	Formula M. Wt	b. p. or m. p. / ℃	Solubility
4'-Azido-3'-O-benzoyl-5'-O-(m-chlorobenzoyl)-2'-deoxy-2'-fluoro-beta-D-arabinouridine (Compound **2**)	1333126-30-9	$C_{23}H_{17}ClFN_5O_7$ 529. 87	—	—
Triazole(Compound **3**)	288-88-0	$C_2H_3N_3$ 69. 07	m. p. 119~121	Well soluble in water; slightly soluble in acetone and ethyl acetate
1-[4-C-Azido-3-O-benzoyl-5-O-(3-chlorobenzoyl)-2-deoxy-2-fluoro-β-D-arabinofuranosyl]-4-(1H-1,2,4-triazol-1-yl)-2(1H)-pyrimidinone(Compound **4**)	1631061-80-7	$C_{25}H_{18}ClFN_8O_6$ 580. 92	m. p. 114~116	—
4-Amino-1-[4-C-azido-3-O-benzoyl-5-O-(3-chlorobenzoyl)-2-deoxy-2-fluoro-β-D-arabinofuranosyl]-2(1H)-pyrimidinone Compound **5**	1596289-91-6	$C_{23}H_{18}ClFN_6O_6$ 528. 88	—	—
Phosphorus oxychloride	$POCl_3$ 10025-87-3	$POCl_3$ 153. 33	b. p. 105. 3	Soluble in many organic solvents
Triethylamine	$C_6H_{15}N$ 86393-33-1	$C_6H_{15}N$ 101. 19	b. p. 90	Slightly soluble in water, the aqueous solution is alkaline
Concentrated ammonia water	$NH_3 \cdot H_2O$ 1336-21-6	$NH_3 \cdot H_2O$ 35. 05	b. p. 37. 7	Well soluble in water
Saturated methanol solution of ammonia	NH_3-MeOH 67-56-1	NH_3-MeOH 32. 04	b. p. 64. 7	Well soluble in water

2. Synthetic route

The synthesis of Azvudine (compound **1**) is carried out using 4′-azido-3′-O-benzoyl-5′-O-(*m*-chlorobenzoyl)-2′-deoxy-2′-fluoro-beta-D-arabinuridine (compound **2**) and triazole (compound **3**) as raw materials. Triazole deoxy substituted bis-benzoyl-uridine (compound **4**) is obtained through a condensation reaction, followed by an aminolysis reaction to obtain bis-benzoyl-protected Azvudine (compound **5**), and finally, the target compound **1** is obtained by debenzoylation.

Safety Tips: Strong acid and alkali reagents such as phosphorus oxychloride and ammonia-methanol will be used in this experiment. Pay attention to ventilation during operation, strictly follow the operating procedures, and wear rubber acid and alkali resistant gloves. Skin is prone to burning when exposed to strong acid and alkali reagents such as phosphorus oxychloride and ammonia-methanol. In cases of mild poisoning, patients can inhale soda vapor, drink mineral water with milk, take expectorants and inducers, and rinse their eyes with a 2% boric acid solution. When the poisoning is severe, it should be promptly taken to the hospital for treatment.

3. Knowledge points

Condensation reaction, ammonolysis reaction, debenzoylation reaction, triazole.

Ⅲ Experimental Equipments and Raw Materials

1. Experimental equipment

The condensation reaction apparatus is composed of a magnetic stirrer, a

The condensation reaction apparatus and the ammonolysis reaction apparatus

three-necked round-bottom flask, a reflux condenser, a constant pressure dropping funnel, an ice-water bath, and a thermometer.

The ammonolysis reaction apparatus is composed of a magnetic stirrer, a three-necked round-bottom flask, a reflux condenser, and a thermometer.

2. Raw materials

Synthetic product	Raw materials			
	Name	Quantity	Quality	Use
Compound **4**	4′-Azido-3′-O-benzoyl-5′-O-(m-chlorobenzoyl)-2′-deoxy-2′-fluoro-beta-D-arabinouridine(Compound **2**)	7.00 g(13.2 mmol)	CP	Reactant
	Triazole(Compound **3**)	8.68 g(125 mmol)	CP	Reactant
	Phosphorus oxychloride	2.54 mL(28 mmol)	CP	Reactant
	Triethylamine	28 mL	CP	Acid-binding agent
	Dichloromethane	150 mL	AR	Solvent
	Distilled water	3 mL	—	Solvent
	Saturated sodium bicarbonate solution	100 mL	Product prepared	Neutralizer
Compound **5**	Compound **4**	3.83 g(6.6 mmol)	Product prepared	Reactant
	Concentrated ammonia water	15 mL	CP	Reactant
	1,4-Dioxane	10 mL	CP	Solvent
Azvudine (Compound **1**)	Compound **5**	3.49 g(6.6 mmol)	Product prepared	Reactant
	Saturated methanol solution of ammonia	10 mL	CP	Reactant
	Dichloromethane	500 mL	CP	Eluent
	Methanol	65 mL	CP	Eluent
	Distilled water	16 mL	—	Solvent

Ⅳ Operations

1. Preparation of compound 4

(1) Equip the condensation reaction apparatus.

(2) In the dry 250 mL three-necked flask, add 8.68 g of triazole (compound **3**) and 100 mL of anhydrous dichloromethane, stir to dissolve, in an ice-water bath, add 2.54 mL of phosphorus oxychloride, and slowly add 17 mL of triethylamine using a constant pressure dropping funnel.

(3) Add 7 g of 4′-azido-3′-O-benzoyl-5′-O-(m-chlorobenzoyl)-2′-deoxy-2′-fluoro-beta-D-arabinouridine (compound **2**).

(4) Remove the ice-water bath, heat to room temperature, and react for 2.5 h.

(5) Slowly add a mixed solution of 3 mL of water and 11 mL of triethylamine, continue stirring for 10 min, then add 100 mL of saturated sodium bicarbonate aqueous solution and 150 mL of dichloromethane, separate the organic layer, and dry with anhydrous sodium sulfate.

(6) Filter and remove the solvent by rotary evaporation to obtain a yellow solid, which can proceed to the next reaction step without further processing.

2. Preparation of compound 5

(1) Equip the ammonolysis reaction apparatus.

(2) In the dry 100 mL three-necked flask, sequentially add the product obtained in the previous step and 10 mL of 1,4-dioxane, stir to dissolve, and then add 15 mL of concentrated ammonia water.

(3) Seal the reaction bottle and continue stirring at room temperature for 5 h.

(4) Remove the solvent from the reaction mixture by rotary evaporation to obtain a reddish-brown viscous substance, which can proceed directly to the next reaction step without further treatment.

3. Preparation of Azvudine (Compound 1)

(1) Equip the ammonolysis reaction apparatus.

(2) In the dry 100 mL three-necked flask, add compound 5 prepared above and 10 mL saturated methanol solution of ammonia. Seal the reaction bottle and stir at room temperature for 8 h.

(3) Add 5 g of silica gel to the reaction mixture, remove the solvent by rotary evaporation, and separate the obtained solid by column chromatography [eluent: dichloromethane-methanol (10 : 1); TLC: dichloromethane-methanol (5 : 1)] to obtain a gray-white solid product (crude Azvudine) .

(4) Add the gray-white solid product obtained above to a 100 mL three-necked flask, then add 16 mL of water and 4 mL of methanol, and heat to 70 ℃ to dissolve the solid.

(5) Filter the obtained hot solution while it is still hot, and allow the filtrate to cool naturally to room temperature for crystallization.

(6) Filter to obtain a light yellow crystalline solid, wash the solid 2~3 times with methanol, dry to obtain Azvudine, weigh it, calculate the yield, and measure the melting point.

(7) Send the final product to the place where the teachers designated.

V Experimental Results

1. Yield

(1) Calculate the theoretical production of Azvudine

$$\text{Compound } \mathbf{2} \quad\text{———}\quad \text{Azvudine}$$
$$M_w - 529.87 \text{ g/mol} \quad\text{———}\quad M_w - 286.22 \text{ g/mol}$$
$$0.0132 \text{ mol} \quad\text{———}\quad 0.0132 \text{ mol}$$

Theoretical production $= 0.0132 \text{ mol} \times 286.22 \text{ g/mol} = 3.87 \text{ g}$

(2) Calculate the percent yield of Azvudine

$$\text{Yield} = \frac{\text{Practical production}}{\text{Theoretical production}} \times 100\% = \frac{(\quad)}{3.87 \text{ g}} \times 100\% = (\quad)\%$$

2. Appearance and melting point of product

A. Appearance: _____ ;

B. m. p. :

Theoretical value: 99～100 ℃;

Practical value: _____.

3. Analysis of experimental results

_____

_____

_____

_____

_____

_____.

Ⅵ Notes

1. Temperature control is an important factor in each step of the reaction.

2. The entire reaction proceeds from the previous step, and the amount of each reagent used needs to be calculated proportionally before use.

Ⅶ Determination of Product Content

Chromatographic conditions: Silica gel matrix reverse phase C_{18} column (3 μm) (150 mm×3 mm) . The mobile phase is a water/acetonitrile solution containing 5 mmol/L ammonium acetate, and the acetonitrile content in the mobile phase changes from 5% to 99% within 3 min. The flow rate is 0.8 mL/min. The injection volume is 5 μL.

Measurement method: High-performance liquid chromatography. Accurately weigh the test sample, dilute it to 100 mL, and prepare the test sample solution. Inject the test solution into the liquid chromatograph, record the chromatogram, and observe the peak of Azvudine at 7.5 min. Calculate the Azvudine content using the peak area normalization method. [Smith D B, Journal of Medicinal Chemistry, 2009, 52 (9): 2971-2978]

Ⅷ Discussion Questions

1. In terms of structure, what other reagents can be used to replace the debenzoylation reaction?

2. In terms of structure, what are the by-products of the debenzoylation reaction during the preparation of Azvudine?

(By Xiaoyu Chang)

实验十八

阿兹夫定的合成

背景知识

　　阿兹夫定（Azvudine，FNC）为病毒逆转录酶抑制剂，为我国拥有自主知识产权的核苷类抗病毒药物，可口服给药，临床用于艾滋病和新冠病毒感染的治疗，阿兹夫定的化学结构如图 18-1 所示。

图 18-1　阿兹夫定的化学结构

阿兹夫定的
作用机制

Ⅰ　目的与要求

　　1. 掌握缩合反应、氨化反应、脱苯甲酰基反应的原理。

　　2. 掌握缩合反应、氨化反应、脱苯甲酰基反应的实验操作。

　　3. 了解阿兹夫定与靶标的作用方式。

Ⅱ　实验原理

1. 主要反应物和产物的物理常数

名称	结构式 CAS 号	分子式 分子量	沸点或 熔点/℃	溶解度
阿兹夫定（化合物 **1**）	1011529-10-4	$C_9H_{11}FN_6O_4$ 286.22	m. p. 99～100	DMSO：57～125 mg/mL； 水：～57 mg/mL；乙醇： ～57 mg/mL

名称	结构式 CAS 号	分子式 分子量	沸点或 熔点/℃	溶解度
4′-叠氮基-3′-O-苯甲酰基-5′-O-(m-氯苯甲酰基)-2′-脱氧-2′-氟-B-D-阿拉伯哌啶（化合物 **2**）	1333126-30-9	$C_{23}H_{17}ClFN_5O_7$ 529.87	—	—
三氮唑（化合物 **3**）	288-88-0	$C_2H_3N_3$ 69.07	m. p. 119~121	易溶于水,微溶于丙酮、乙酸乙酯
1-[4-C-叠氮基-3-O-苯甲酰基-5-O-(3-氯苯甲酰基)-2-脱氧-2-氟-β-D-阿拉伯呋喃糖基]-4-(1H-1,2,4-三唑-1-基)-2(1H)-嘧啶酮（化合物 **4**）	1631061-80-7	$C_{25}H_{18}ClFN_8O_6$ 580.92	m. p. 114~116	
氨基-1-[4-C-叠氮基-3-O-苯甲酰基-5-O-(3-氯苯甲酰基)-2-脱氧-2-氟-β-D-阿拉伯呋喃糖基]-2(1H)-嘧啶酮（化合物 **5**）	1596289-91-6	$C_{23}H_{18}ClFN_6O_6$ 528.88	—	—
三氯氧磷	$POCl_3$ 10025-87-3	$POCl_3$ 153.33	b. p. 105.3	可溶于许多有机溶剂
三乙胺	$C_6H_{15}N$ 86393-33-1	$C_6H_{15}N$ 101.19	b. p. 90	微溶于水,水溶液呈碱性
浓氨水	$NH_3 \cdot H_2O$ 1336-21-6	$NH_3 \cdot H_2O$ 35.05	b. p. 37.7	易溶于水
氨的甲醇饱和溶液	NH_3-MeOH 67-56-1	NH_3-MeOH 32.04	b. p. 64.7	易溶于水

2. 合成路线

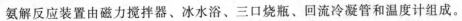

阿兹夫定（化合物 **1**）的合成以 4′-叠氮基-3′-O-苯甲酰基-5′-O-(m-氯苯甲酰基)-2′-脱氧-2′-氟-B-D-阿拉伯哌啶（化合物 **2**）和三氮唑（化合物 **3**）为原料，经缩合反应获得三氮唑脱氧取代双苯甲酰基尿苷（化合物 **4**），再经氨解反应获得双苯甲酰基保护的阿兹夫定（化合物 **5**），最后脱苯甲酰基得到目标化合物 **1**。

安全提示：本实验中会用到三氯氧磷、氨-甲醇等强酸强碱试剂，在操作中注意通风，严格遵守操作规程，戴橡胶耐酸碱手套。皮肤与三氯氧磷、氨-甲醇等强酸强碱试剂接触容易灼伤，轻度中毒时可给患者吸苏打蒸气、喝加牛奶的矿泉水、服祛痰剂及诱导剂，用 2% 的硼酸溶液冲洗眼睛。中毒较重时应速送医院治疗。

3. 知识点

缩合反应，氨解反应，脱苯甲酰基反应，三氮唑。

Ⅲ 实验装置和原料

1. 实验装置

缩合反应装置由磁力搅拌器、三口烧瓶、回流冷凝管、恒压滴液漏斗、冰水浴和温度计组成。

氨解反应装置由磁力搅拌器、冰水浴、三口烧瓶、回流冷凝管和温度计组成。

缩合反应
装置和氨解
反应装置

2. 原料

合成产物	原料			
	名称	用量	试剂级别	用途
化合物 **4**	4′-叠氮基-3′-O-苯甲酰基-5′-O-(m-氯苯甲酰基)-2′-脱氧-2′-氟-B-D-阿拉伯哌啶（化合物 **2**）	7.00 g（13.2 mmol）	化学纯	反应物
	三氮唑（化合物 **3**）	8.68 g（125 mmol）	化学纯	反应物

合成产物	原料			
	名称	用量	试剂级别	用途
化合物 4	三氯氧磷	2.54 mL(28 mmol)	化学纯	反应物
	三乙胺	28 mL	化学纯	缚酸剂
	二氯甲烷	150 mL	分析纯	溶剂
	蒸馏水	3 mL	—	溶剂
	饱和碳酸氢钠	100 mL	自制	中和剂
化合物 5	化合物 4	3.83 g(6.6 mmol)	自制	反应物
	浓氨水	15 mL	化学纯	反应物
	1,4-二氧六环	10 mL	化学纯	溶剂
阿兹夫定 (化合物 1)	化合物 5	3.49 g(6.6 mmol)	自制	反应物
	氨的甲醇饱和溶液	10 mL	化学纯	反应物
	二氯甲烷	500 mL	化学纯	洗脱剂
	甲醇	65 mL	化学纯	洗脱剂
	蒸馏水	16 mL	—	溶剂

Ⅳ 实验操作

1. 化合物 4 的制备

(1) 搭建缩合反应装置。

(2) 在干燥的 250 mL 三口烧瓶中，加入 8.68 g 三氮唑（化合物 3）和 100 mL 无水二氯甲烷，搅拌溶解后，冰水浴下加入 2.54 mL 三氯氧磷，再用恒压滴液漏斗慢慢滴加 17 mL 三乙胺。

(3) 加入 7 g 4′-叠氮基-3′-O-苯甲酰基-5′-O-(m-氯苯甲酰基)-2′-脱氧-2′-氟-β-D-阿拉伯哌啶（化合物 2）。

(4) 撤去冰水浴，升温至室温，反应 2.5 h。

(5) 慢慢加入 3 mL 水和 11 mL 三乙胺的混合溶液，继续搅拌反应 10 min 后，加入 100 mL 饱和碳酸氢钠水溶液和 150 mL 二氯甲烷，分出有机相，无水硫酸钠干燥。

(6) 过滤，旋转蒸发除去溶剂，得到黄色固体，无需进一步处理可直接进行下一步反应。

2. 化合物 5 的制备

(1) 搭建氨解反应装置。

(2) 在干燥的 100 mL 三口烧瓶中，依次加入 10 mL 1,4-二氧六环和上步所得产品，搅拌溶解后再加入 15 mL 浓氨水。

(3) 密封反应瓶，室温下继续搅拌 5 h。

(4) 将反应混合液旋转蒸发除去溶剂，得红棕色黏稠物，无需进一步处理可直接进行下一步反应。

3. 阿兹夫定（化合物 1）的制备

(1) 搭建氨解反应装置。

（2）在干燥的 100 mL 三口烧瓶中，加入上步制备的化合物 **5**、10 mL 氨的甲醇饱和溶液。密封反应瓶，室温下搅拌 8 h。

（3）向反应混合物中加入 5 g 硅胶，旋转蒸发除去溶剂，将所得固体进行柱色谱分离（洗脱剂：二氯甲烷-甲醇＝10∶1；TLC：二氯甲烷-甲醇＝5∶1），得灰白色固体产品（阿兹夫定粗品）。

（4）将获得的灰白色固体产品加入到 100 mL 三口烧瓶中，再加入 16 mL 水和 4 mL 甲醇，加热至 70 ℃使固体溶解。

（5）将所得热溶液趁热过滤，滤液自然冷却至室温，析晶。

（6）抽滤得到淡黄色晶状固体，用甲醇洗涤固体 2～3 次，干燥得阿兹夫定，称重，计算收率，测熔点。

（7）将产物送到指导教师指定的产品回收处。

V 实验结果

1. 收率

（1）计算阿兹夫定的理论产量。

$$化合物 \textbf{2} \text{————} 阿兹夫定$$
$$M_w = 529.87\ g/mol \text{————} M_w = 286.22\ g/mol$$
$$0.0132\ mol \text{————} 0.0132\ mol$$

理论产量＝0.0132 mol×286.22 g/mol＝3.78 g

（2）计算阿兹夫定的收率

$$收率 = \frac{产品实际产量}{产品理论产量} \times 100\% = \frac{(\quad\quad)}{3.78\ g} \times 100\% = (\quad\quad)\%$$

2. 产品外观与熔点

A. 外观：＿＿＿＿＿＿＿＿＿＿＿＿＿＿＿＿＿＿＿＿＿；

B. 熔点：

　　理论值：99～100 ℃；

　　实测值：＿＿＿＿＿＿＿＿＿＿＿＿＿＿＿＿＿。

3. 实验结果分析

＿＿＿＿＿＿＿＿＿＿＿＿＿＿＿＿＿＿＿＿＿＿＿＿＿＿＿＿＿＿＿＿＿＿＿＿＿＿

＿＿＿＿＿＿＿＿＿＿＿＿＿＿＿＿＿＿＿＿＿＿＿＿＿＿＿＿＿＿＿＿＿＿＿＿＿＿

＿＿＿＿＿＿＿＿＿＿＿＿＿＿＿＿＿＿＿＿＿＿＿＿＿＿＿＿＿＿＿＿＿＿＿＿＿＿

＿＿＿＿＿＿＿＿＿＿＿＿＿＿＿＿＿＿＿＿＿＿＿＿＿＿＿＿＿＿＿＿＿＿＿＿＿＿

＿＿＿＿＿＿＿＿＿＿＿＿＿＿＿＿＿＿＿＿＿＿＿＿＿＿＿＿＿＿＿＿＿＿＿＿＿＿

＿＿＿＿＿＿＿＿＿＿＿＿＿＿＿＿＿＿＿＿＿＿＿＿＿＿＿＿＿＿＿＿＿＿＿＿＿＿

＿＿＿＿＿＿＿＿＿＿＿＿＿＿＿＿＿＿＿＿＿＿＿＿＿＿＿＿＿＿＿＿＿＿＿＿＿＿。

VI 注意事项

1. 各步骤反应温度控制是重要的因素。

2. 整个反应是接着上一步反应进行的，所用试剂的量需要按照比例计算后使用。

Ⅶ 产物的含量测定

色谱条件：硅胶基质反相 C_{18} 色谱柱（$3\,\mu m$）（$150\,mm \times 3\,mm$）；流动相为 A 为含有 $5\,mmol/L$ 乙酸铵的水/乙腈溶液，3 分钟内流动相中乙腈含量从 5% 转变为 99%；流速为 $0.8\,mL/min$；进样量为 $5\,\mu L$。

测定法：高效液相色谱法。精密称定供试品，稀释至 $100\,mL$，配置成供试品溶液。将供试品溶液注入液相色谱仪，记录色谱图，阿兹夫定在 $7.5\,min$ 出峰，按照峰面积归一法计算阿兹夫定含量。［Smith D B，Journal of Medicinal Chemistry，2009，52（9）：2971-2978］

Ⅷ 思考题

1. 用结构式表示，脱苯甲酰基反应还可以用什么试剂代替？
2. 用结构式表示，阿兹夫定制备时脱苯甲酰基反应的副产物是什么？

（常晓宇）

Experiment 19

Synthesis of Olverembatinib

Background

Olverembatinib is a novel anticancer drug targeting the Abl kinase, which was designed and developed by scientists in China, approved for the treatment of adult patients with TKI-resistant chronic-phase chronic myeloid leukaemia (CML) or accelerated-phase CML harbouring the T315I mutation. The chemical structure of olverembatinib is illustrated in Fig. 19-1.

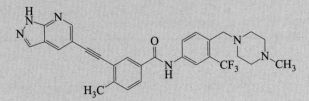

The mechanism of action of Olverembatinib

Fig. 19-1　Chemical structure of Olverembatinib.

Ⅰ Purposes and Requirements

1. To master the principle of aminolysis of esters and Sonogashira coupling reaction.

2. To master the reaction operation of aminolysis of esters and Sonogashira coupling reaction.

3. To understand the mode of action of Olverembatinib and Bcr-Abl.

Ⅱ Principle of the Reaction

1. Physical data of the main reactants and product

Name	Structure CAS No.	Formula M. Wt	b. p. or m. p. / ℃	Solubility
Olverembatinib (Compound 1)	 1257628-77-5	$C_{29}H_{27}F_3N_6O$ 532. 56	b. p. 630. 4±55. 0	DMSO：≥100 mg/mL(187. 77 mmol/L)

Name	Structure / CAS No.	Formula / M. Wt	b. p. or m. p. / ℃	Solubility
Methyl 3-iodo-4-methylbenzoat (Compound **2**)	H_3C, I, CH_3 90347-66-3	$C_9H_9IO_2$ 276.07	b. p. 302.9 ± 30.0	Not miscible or difficult to mix with water
4-(4-Methylpiperazinomethyl)-3-(trifluoromethyl)aniline (Compound **3**)	CH_3 ... F_3C, NH_2 694499-26-8	$C_{13}H_{18}F_3N_3$ 273.30	b. p. 329.1 ± 42.0	—
3-Iodo-4-methyl-N-(4-((4-methylpiperazin-1-yl)methyl)-3-(trifluoromethyl)phenyl)benzamide (Compound **4**)	CH_3 ... F_3C, NH, O, I, CH_3 943320-50-1	$C_{21}H_{23}F_3IN_3O$ 517.33	b. p. 466.6 ± 45.0	—
5-Ethynyl-1H-pyrazolo[3,4-b]pyridine (Compound **5**)	H, N, N, CH 1207351-15-2	$C_8H_5N_3$ 143.15	b. p. 335.7 ± 22.0	—
Potassium *tert*-butoxide	*t*-BuOK 865-47-4	C_4H_9OK 112.21	m. p. $256\sim258$	Soluble in hexane, toluene, diethyl ether, and tetrahydrofuran
Bis(triphenylphosphine)palladium(Ⅱ)dichloride	$Pd(PPh_3)_2Cl_2$ 13965-03-2	$C_{36}H_{30}Cl_2P_2Pd$ 701.9	m. p. 260	Insoluble in water. Soluble in benzene, and toluene
Cuprous iodide	CuI 7681-65-4	CuI 190.45	m. p. 605	Dilute acidic aqueous solution; insoluble (upon heating)
Triethylamine	Et_3N 121-44-8	$C_6H_{15}N$ 101.19	b. p. 90	Water: soluble up to 112 g/L at 20 ℃
Tetrahydrofuran	THF 109-99-9	C_4H_8O 72.11	b. p. 66	Easy to soluble in water
Acetonitrile	CH_3CN 75-05-8	C_2H_3N 41.05	b. p. $81\sim82$	Soluble in many organic solvents

2. Synthetic route

The synthesis of Olverembatinib initiates with methyl 3-iodo-4-methylbenzoat (compound **2**) and 4-(4-methylpiperazinomethyl)-3-(trifluoromethyl) aniline (compound **3**). These starting materials undergo an aminolysis of ester under basic conditions to obtain 3-iodo-4-methyl-*N*-(4-((4-methylpiperazin-1-yl) methyl)-3-(trifluoromethyl) phenyl) benzamide (compound **4**). Then, coupling of 5-ethynyl-1*H*-pyrazolo［3, 5-ethynyl-1*H*-pyrazolo［3, 4-b］ pyridine (compound **5**) with aromatic iodide **4** through palladium-catalyzed Sonogashira coupling reaction yielded the desired inhibitor Olvermbatinib.

Safety Tips: During the experiment, the strong base potassium *tert*-butoxide must be handled with caution. It is crucial to prevent any contact with water or acidic substances to prevent vigorous reactions. Furthermore, due to its sensitivity to air and moisture, it should be manipulated in an inert atmosphere and stored in a dry, sealed container to ensure its stability and reactivity.

3. Knowledge points

Aminolysis of esters reaction, Sonogashira coupling reaction, potassium *tert*-butoxide.

Ⅲ Experimental Equipments and Raw Materials

1. Experimental equipment

The aminolysis reaction apparatus is composed of a magnetic stirrer, a three-necked round-bottom flask, a reflux condenser, a constant pressure dropping funnel, an ice-salt bath, and a thermometer.

The Sonogashira coupling reaction apparatus is composed of a magnetic stir-

The aminolysis reaction apparatus and the Sonogashira coupling reaction apparatus

rer, a three-neck round-bottom flask, a reflux condenser, a balloon filled with argon gas, a glass T connector tube, and a thermometer.

2. Raw materials

Synthetic product	Raw materials			
	Name	Quantity	Name	Use
Compound **4**	Methyl 3-iodo-4-methylbenzoat (Compound **2**)	8. 6 g (31. 16 mmol)	CP	Reactant
	4-(4-Methylpiperazinomethyl)-3-(trifluoromethyl)aniline (Compound **3**)	8. 5 g (31. 16 mmol)	CP	Reactant
	Potassium *tert*-butoxide	21. 0 g (186. 96 mmol)	CP	Base
	Tetrahydrofuran	150 mL	AR	Solvent
Olverembatinib (Compound **1**)	Compound **4**	2. 6 g (5. 0 mmol)	Product prepared	Reactant
	5-Ethynyl-1*H*-pyrazolo[3,5-ethynyl-1*H*-pyrazolo[3,4-b]pyridine (Compound **5**)	0. 72 g (5. 0 mmol)	CP	Reactant
	Bis(triphenylphosphine)palladium(Ⅱ)dichloride	350 mg (0. 5 mmol)	CP	Catalyst
	Cuprous iodide	95 mg (0. 5 mmol)	CP	Catalyst
	Triethylamine	2. 1 mL (15. 0 mmol)	CP	Base
	Acetonitrile	50 mL	AR	Solvent
	Dichloromethane	800 mL	AR	Solvent
	Methanol	100 mL	AR	Solvent

Ⅳ Operations

1. Preparation of compound 4

(1) Equip the aminolysis reaction apparatus.

(2) In the 250 mL three-necked flask, add 8. 6 g of methyl 3-iodo-4-methylbenzoate (compound **2**), 8. 5 g of 3-(trifluoromethyl)-4-[(4-methylpiperazin-1-yl) methyl] aniline (compound **3**), and 100 mL of THF. Stir to dissolve, then cool the mixture to $-20\ ℃$.

(3) Dissolve 21. 0 g of *t*-BuOK in 50 mL of THF and slowly add it to the mixture using a dropping funnel. Stirring at $-20\ ℃$ for 1 h, then raise to room temperature and react for another 2 h.

(4) Pour the reaction mixture slowly into 1 L of water, then let it stand overnight.

(5) Filter the precipitated solid, wash it with water, and dry it to obtain the crude product. Use the product directly for the next reaction step.

2. Preparation of Olverembatinib (Compound 1)

(1) Equip the Sonogashira reaction apparatus.

(2) Under argon, add 2. 6 g of compound **4**, 0. 72 g of 5-ethynyl-1*H*-pyrazolo[3,4-b] pyridine (compound **5**), and 50 mL of dry CH_3CN to a dry 100 mL three-neck flask. Stir to mix, then add 350 mg of $Pd(PPh_3)_2Cl_2$, 95 mg of CuI, and 2. 1 mL of Et_3N.

(3) Heat to 100 ℃ and stir under argon for about 20 h.

(4) After the reaction is complete, cool to room temperature and filter.

(5) Add silica gel to the filtrate, remove the solvent by rotary evaporation, and then separate the solid obtained by column chromatography (eluent: dichloromethane-methanol) to yield a gray to yellow solid product.

(6) Send the final product to the place where the teachers designated.

V Experimental Results

1. Yield

(1) Calculate the theoretical production of Olverembatinib

$$\text{Compound } \mathbf{2} \text{———— Olverembatinib}$$
$$M_w = 276.07 \text{ g/mol} \text{————} M_w = 532.56 \text{ g/mol}$$
$$0.0312 \text{ mol} \text{————} 0.0312 \text{ mol}$$
$$\text{Theoretical production} = 0.0312 \text{ mol} \times 532.56 \text{ g/mol} = 16.62 \text{ g}$$

(2) Calculate the percent yield of Olverembatinib

$$\text{Yield} = \frac{\text{Practical production}}{\text{Theoretical production}} \times 100\% = \frac{(\qquad)}{16.62 \text{ g}} \times 100\% = (\qquad)\%$$

2. Appearance and melting point of product

A. Appearance: _____ ;

B. m. p. :

Theoretical value: 232~234 ℃ ;

Practical value: _____ .

3. Analysis of experimental results

_____

_____

_____

_____

_____

_____

_____ .

VI Notes

1. In the post-treatment process of compound **4**, pay attention to the complete separation and washing of the solid during filtration and water washing to minimize the introduction of impurities.

2. For the aminolysis reaction of compound **4** and the Sonogashira coupling reaction of compound **1**, it is necessary to strictly control the reaction temperature and time. Particularly for the Sonogashira coupling reaction, it must be conducted under argon protection, as an oxygen-free environment is crucial for the palladium catalyst to exert its catalytic effect.

3. The entire reaction proceeds from the previous step, and the amounts of reagents used must be calculated proportionally.

Ⅶ Discussion Questions

1. What are some other methods for the synthesis of amide groups?

2. During the synthesis of Olverembatinib, consider what factors might affect the efficiency of the Sonogashira coupling reaction and propose possible optimization strategies.

(By Xiaoyun Lu)

实验十九

奥雷巴替尼的合成

背景知识

奥雷巴替尼（Olverembatinib）是以 Abelson 酪氨酸激酶（Abelson tyrosine kinase，Abl）为靶标的新型抗肿瘤药物，是我国研发的原创新药，适用于任何酪氨酸激酶抑制剂耐药，并伴有 breakpoint cluster region-Abl Thr315Ile（Bcr-Abl[T315I]）突变的慢性髓细胞白血病慢性期或加速期的成年患者。奥雷巴替尼的化学结构如图 19-1 所示。

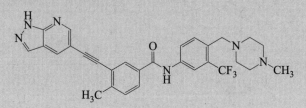

图 19-1 奥雷巴替尼的化学结构

奥雷巴替尼的作用机制

I 目的与要求

1. 掌握酯的氨解和 Sonogashira 偶联反应的原理。
2. 掌握酯的氨解和 Sonogashira 偶联反应的实验操作。
3. 了解奥雷巴替尼与激酶的结合模式。

II 实验原理

1. 主要反应物和产物的物理常数

名称	结构式 CAS 号	分子式 分子量	沸点或 熔点/℃	溶解度
奥雷巴替尼 （化合物 1）	1257628-77-5	$C_{29}H_{27}F_3N_6O$ 532.56	b. p. 630.4±55.0	二甲基亚砜：≥100 mg/mL(187.77 mmol/L)

名称	结构式 CAS 号	分子式 分子量	沸点或 熔点/℃	溶解度
3-碘-4-甲基苯甲酸 甲酯(化合物 **2**)	 90347-66-3	$C_9H_9IO_2$ 276.07	b. p. 302.9±30.0	不能与水混 溶或难以与水 混溶
3-三氟甲基-4- [(4-甲基哌嗪-1-基) 甲基]苯胺(化合物 **3**)	 694499-26-8	$C_{13}H_{18}F_3N_3$ 273.30	b. p. 329.1±42.0	—
3-碘-4-甲基-*N*- [4-[(4-甲基-1-哌嗪基) 甲基]-3-(三氟甲基) 苯基]苯甲酰胺 (化合物 **4**)	 943320-50-1	$C_{21}H_{23}F_3IN_3O$ 517.33	b. p. 466.6±45.0	—
5-乙炔基-1*H*-吡唑 并[3,4-B]吡啶 (化合物 **5**)	 1207351-15-2	$C_8H_5N_3$ 143.15	b. p. 335.7±22.0	—
叔丁醇钾	*t*-BuOK 865-47-4	C_4H_9KO 112.21	m. p. 256~258	溶于己烷、 甲苯、乙醚和 四氢呋喃
双三苯基磷 二氯化钯	$Pd(PPh_3)_2Cl_2$ 13965-03-2	$C_{36}H_{30}Cl_2P_2Pd$ 701.9	m. p. 260	不溶于水, 溶于苯和甲苯
碘化亚铜	CuI 7681-65-4	CuI 190.45	m. p. 605	稀酸水溶 液:不溶(加 热)
三乙胺	Et_3N 121-44-8	$C_6H_{15}N$ 101.19	b. p. 90	水:112 g/L (20 ℃)
四氢呋喃	THF 109-99-9	C_4H_8O 72.11	b. p. 66	可溶于水
乙腈	CH_3CN 75-05-8	C_2H_3N 41.05	b. p. 81~82	溶于有机溶 剂

2. 合成路线

H₃C, I, OCH₃ — 2 + 3 (N-methylpiperazine aniline) → *t*-BuOK / THF, −20 ℃ to r.t. → 4

5-ethynyl pyrazolopyridine — 5

Pd(PPh₃)₂Cl₂, CuI, Et₃N
ACN, 100 ℃ , argon → 1

奥雷巴替尼（化合物 **1**）的合成以 3-碘-4-甲基苯甲酸甲酯（化合物 **2**）和 3-三氟甲基-4-［(4-甲基哌嗪-1-基)甲基］苯胺（化合物 **3**）为起始原料，在碱性条件下经酯的氨解得到关键中间体 3-碘-4-甲基-N-［4-［(4-甲基-1-哌嗪基)甲基］-3-(三氟甲基)苯基］苯甲酰胺（化合物 **4**），化合物 **4** 再与 5-乙炔基-1*H*-吡唑并［3,4-B］吡啶（化合物 **5**）发生 Sonogashira 偶联反应得到目标化合物 **1**。

安全提示：本实验需要使用强碱试剂叔丁醇钾，在处理时需要小心，避免与水或酸性物质接触，以防止剧烈反应。此外，叔丁醇钾对空气和湿气敏感，应在惰性气体氛围下使用，并储存于干燥、密封的容器中。

3. 知识点

酯的氨解反应，Sonogashira 偶联反应，叔丁醇钾。

酯的氨解
反应装置和
Sonogashira
偶联反应装置

Ⅲ 实验装置和原料

1. 实验装置

酯的氨解反应装置由磁力搅拌器、三口烧瓶、回流冷凝管、恒压滴液漏斗、冰盐浴和温度计组成。

Sonogashira 偶联反应装置由磁力搅拌器、三口烧瓶、球形冷凝管、装有氩气的气球、玻璃三通接头和温度计组成。

2. 原料

合成产物	原料			
	名称	用量	试剂级别	用途
化合物 4	3-碘-4-甲基苯甲酸甲酯(化合物 2)	8.6 g(31.16 mmol)	化学纯	反应物
	3-三氟甲基-4-[(4-甲基哌嗪-1-基)甲基]苯胺(化合物 3)	8.5 g(31.16 mmol)	化学纯	反应物
	叔丁醇钾	21.0 g(186.96 mmol)	化学纯	碱
	四氢呋喃	150 mL	分析纯	溶剂

合成产物	原料			
	名称	用量	试剂级别	用途
奥雷巴替尼 （化合物 1）	化合物 4	2.6 g(5.0 mmol)	自制	反应物
	5-乙炔基-1*H*-吡唑并[3,4-B]吡啶（化合物 5）	0.72 g(5.0 mmol)	化学纯	反应物
	双三苯基磷二氯化钯	350 mg(0.5 mmol)	化学纯	催化剂
	碘化亚铜	95 mg(0.5 mmol)	化学纯	催化剂
	三乙胺	2.1 mL(15.0 mmol)	化学纯	碱
	乙腈	50 mL	分析纯	溶剂
	二氯甲烷	800 mL	分析纯	洗脱剂
	甲醇	100 mL	分析纯	洗脱剂

Ⅳ 实验操作

1. 化合物 4 的制备

（1）搭建酯的氨解反应装置。

（2）在干燥的 250 mL 三口烧瓶中加入 8.6 g 3-碘-4-甲基苯甲酸甲酯（化合物 **2**）、8.5 g 3-三氟甲基-4-[(4-甲基哌嗪-1-基)甲基]苯胺（化合物 **3**）和 100 mL 四氢呋喃，搅拌溶解，并将体系降温至 $-20\ ℃$。

（3）将 21.0 g 叔丁醇钾溶于 50 mL 四氢呋喃中，利用滴液漏斗缓慢滴加至前述混合液中，滴加完毕后维持 $-20\ ℃$ 搅拌 1 h，然后缓慢升至室温继续搅拌 2 h。

（4）在搅拌下将上述反应体系缓慢倒入 1 L 水中，静置过夜。

（5）将析出的固体抽滤，水洗，干燥，得粗品，将粗品直接用于下一步反应。

2. 奥雷巴替尼（化合物 1）的制备

（1）搭建 Sonogashira 偶联反应装置。

（2）氩气氛围保护下，在干燥的 100 mL 三口烧瓶中加入 2.6 g 化合物 **4**、0.72 g 5-乙炔基-1*H*-吡唑并[3,4-B]吡啶（化合物 **5**）和 50 mL 干燥的乙腈，搅拌使混合均匀后，继续加入 350 mg 双三苯基磷二氯化钯、95 mg 碘化亚铜和 2.1 mL 三乙胺。

（3）升温至 100 ℃，在氩气保护下搅拌约 20 h。

（4）反应完毕后，冷却至室温，抽滤。

（5）滤液中加入硅胶，旋转蒸发除去溶剂，将所得固体进行柱色谱分离（洗脱剂：二氯甲烷-甲醇），得灰白色至黄色固体产品。

（6）将产物送到指导教师指定的产品回收处。

Ⅴ 实验结果

1. 收率

（1）计算奥雷巴替尼的理论产量。

$$化合物\ 2\ \text{————}\ 奥雷巴替尼$$
$$M_w=276.07\ g/mol\ \text{————}\ M_w=532.56\ g/mol$$
$$0.0312\ mol\ \text{————}\ 0.0312\ mol$$
$$理论产量=0.0312\ mol\times532.56\ g/mol=16.62\ g$$

（2）计算奥雷巴替尼的收率

$$收率 = \frac{产品实际产量}{产品理论产量} \times 100\% = \frac{(\qquad)}{16.62\text{ g}} \times 100\% = (\qquad)\%$$

2. 产品外观与熔点

A. 外观：_____；

B. 熔点：

理论值：232～234 ℃；

实测值：_____。

3. 实验结果分析

_____

_____

_____

_____

_____

_____

_____。

Ⅵ 注意事项

1. 在化合物 **4** 的后处理过程中，抽滤和水洗时要注意固体的完全分离和洗涤，以减少杂质的引入。

2. 在进行化合物 **4** 的氨解反应和化合物 **1** 的 Sonogashira 偶联反应时，需要严格控制反应温度和时间。特别是 Sonogashira 偶联反应，需要在氩气保护下进行，无氧环境是钯催化剂发挥催化作用的关键。

3. 整个反应是接着上一步反应进行的，所用试剂的量需按照比例计算后使用。

Ⅶ 思考题

1. 还有哪些方法可以合成酰胺基团？

2. 在合成奥雷巴替尼的过程中，考虑哪些因素可能影响 Sonogashira 偶联反应的效率，并提出可能的优化策略。

（陆小云）

Appendix 1　Experimental Report Template

Experiment 2　Synthesis of Aspirin

Ⅰ　Objectives of this Experiment

1. To master the acetylation reaction and its use in structural modification of drug substances.

2. To master the anhydrous operation method，and the use of coloration reaction on the endpoint deterction of organic synthesis.

3. To understand the interaction between aspirin and target.

Ⅱ　Principle of the Reaction

$$\text{Salicylic acid} + \text{Acetic anhydride} \xrightarrow{H_2SO_4} \text{Aspirin} + CH_3COOH$$

Salicylic acid　　Acetic anhydride　　　　　Aspirin　　　Acetic acid

Ⅲ　Experimental Equipments and Raw Materials

1. Experimental equipment

The reflux setup （Fig. 2-1），is composed of a three-neck round-bottom flask，a condenser，a magnetic stirrer，and a thermometer.

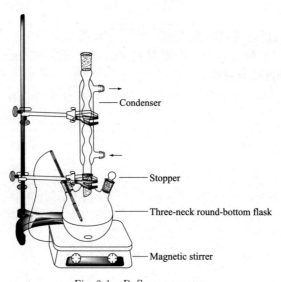

Fig. 2-1　Reflux apparatus

2. Raw materials

Different raw materials will be used in this experiment. They are:

Name	Quantity	Quality	Use
Salicyclic acid	8. 3 g (0. 06 mol)	CP	Reactant
Acetic anhydride	15 mL (0. 159 mol)	CP	Acetylating agent
Sulfuric acid	0. 4 mL (5 drops)	CP	Catalyst
Ethanol	12 mL	95 %	Solvent for recryst
$FeCl_3$ reagent	1 drop	—	Endpoint measurement
Na_2CO_3	10 mL	—	Hydrolysing agent
H_2SO_4 diluted	10 mL	—	Neutralizing agent
Active carbon(Charcoal)	0. 5 g	—	Decolorizing substance

IV Operations

Creat a data table to record the necessary quantitative information for this lab, as well as your observations of what occurred.

No.	Experimental operation	Experimental phenomena	Phenomena explanation
1	Take 15 mL of acetic acid anhydride and 5 drops of concentrated sulfuric acid and place them in 100 mL three-neck round-bottom flask. Assemble the reflux apparatus (as Fig. 2-1). Agitate gently; in parallel, raising the temperature at 55~60 ℃ on the steam bath.	It took five minutes to rise temperature from room to 55~60 ℃.	At the beginning of the reaction, it is necessary to slowly heat to avoid the occurrence of side reactions caused by violent reactions.
2	Add 8. 3 g of salicylic acid crystals to the reaction mixture; dissolve them and keep at 55~60 ℃.	It took 15 minutes to dissolve, and a colorless clarifying solution was obtained.	Salicylic acid reacts with acetic anhydride to form acetylsalicylic acid.
3	...	...	...
4	...	...	...
5	...	...	...

V Experimental Results

1. Yield

$$\text{Yield} = \frac{\text{Practical production}}{\text{Theoretical production}} \times 100\% = \frac{(\quad)}{10.\ 81\ g} \times 100\% = (\quad)\%$$

2. Appearance and melting point of product

A. Appearance: _____ ;

B. m. p. :

　　Theoretical value: 135~138 ℃;

Practical value: _____ 。

3. Analysis of experimental results

The yield of aspirin in this experiment is 60 %. Although the yield is considerable, there are still possibilities for further improvement, such as: ①washing flasks with a small amount of solvent to collect product when the reaction solution is transferred; ②thermal filtration is faster during recrystallization operation; ③the amount of recrystallization solvent should be controlled as much as possible in just dissolving solids. The melting range of the product is short and the value is in accordance with the theoretical value. It shows that the content of the product is high. The structure of the product can be further confirmed by NMR, MS, IR and elemental analysis. The content of the product can be further confirmed by high performance solution chromatography (HPLC).

Ⅵ Discussion Questions

1. In terms of structure, why does/might our room smell like vinegar during this experiment?

2. In terms of structure, why are salicyclic and acetylsalicylic acid considered as acids?

Salicylic acid

Aspirin[2- (acetyloxy) -benzoic acid]

附录一　实验报告模板

实验二　阿司匹林的合成

Ⅰ　实验目的

1. 掌握酯化反应原理和其在药物结构改造中的应用。
2. 掌握无水反应操作；掌握颜色反应在反应终点判断方面的应用。
3. 了解阿司匹林与靶标的作用方式。

Ⅱ　实验原理

水杨酸　　　　　　乙酸酐　　$\xrightarrow{H_2SO_4}$　　阿司匹林　　　+　CH_3COOH

水杨酸　　　　　　　　乙酸酐　　　　　　　　　阿司匹林　　　　　　醋酸

Ⅲ　实验装置和原料

1. 实验装置

反应装置如图 2-1 所示，主要由三口烧瓶、回流冷凝管、磁力搅拌器、温度计组成。

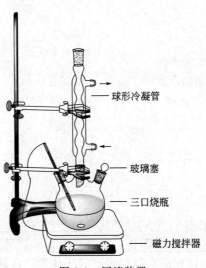

　　　　　　　球形冷凝管

　　　　　　　玻璃塞

　　　　　　　三口烧瓶

　　　　　　　磁力搅拌器

图 2-1　回流装置

2. 原料

名称	用量	试剂级别	用途
水杨酸	8.3 g(0.06 mol)	化学纯	反应物
乙酸酐	15 mL(0.159 mol)	化学纯	酰化试剂
浓硫酸	0.4 mL(5 drops)	化学纯	催化剂
乙醇	12 mL	95 %	重结晶溶剂
$FeCl_3$ 试液	1 drop	—	终点指示剂
Na_2CO_3	10 mL	—	水解剂
稀 H_2SO_4	10 mL	—	中和试剂
活性炭	0.5 g	—	脱色剂

Ⅳ 实验过程

合成和分离（列表，翔实记录实验现象）

步骤	实验操作	实验现象	现象解释
1	搭建反应装置。在 100 mL 三口烧瓶中，加入 15 mL 乙酸酐和 5 滴浓硫酸，搅拌状态下，升温至 55～60 ℃	从室温升高到 55～60 ℃用了 5 min	反应初期，需要缓慢升温，以避免剧烈反应导致副反应的发生
2	在以上体系中，加入 8.3 g 水杨酸晶体，55～60℃下搅拌溶解，可观察到白色晶体逐渐溶解	搅拌溶解用了 15 min，得到无色澄清溶液	水杨酸与乙酸酐发生反应，生成了乙酰水杨酸
3	…	…	…
4	…	…	…
5	…	…	…

Ⅴ 实验结果

1. 收率

$$收率 = \frac{产品实际产量}{产品理论产量} \times 100\% = \frac{(\quad)}{10.8\,g} \times 100\% = (\qquad)\%$$

2. 产品外观与熔点

A. 外观：_____；

B. 熔点：

理论值：135～138 ℃；

实测值：_____。

3. 实验结果分析

本实验中阿司匹林的收率为 60 %，虽然收率较为可观，但是，仍有进一步提高的可能，如①反应液转移时，用少量溶剂洗涤烧瓶，以收集产品；②重结晶操作时，热过滤更为迅速；③重结晶溶剂的用量尽可能控制在能恰好溶解固体等。所测得的产品的熔程较短，数值与理论值相符，说明产品含量较高，进一步确证产物结构，可采用核磁共振（NMR）、质谱（MS）、红外光谱（IR）和元素分析进行分析，进一步确证产物含量，可采用高效液相色谱

（HPLC）进行分析。

VI 思考题

1. 用结构式表示，为什么在反应过程中室内会有醋酸的味道？

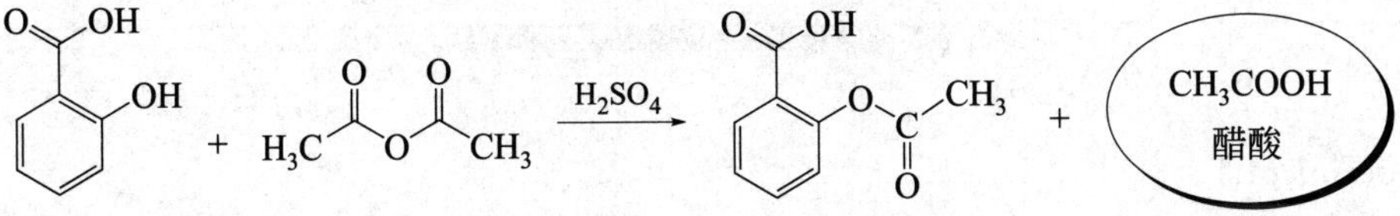

2. 用结构式表示，为什么水杨酸和阿司匹林是酸性物质？

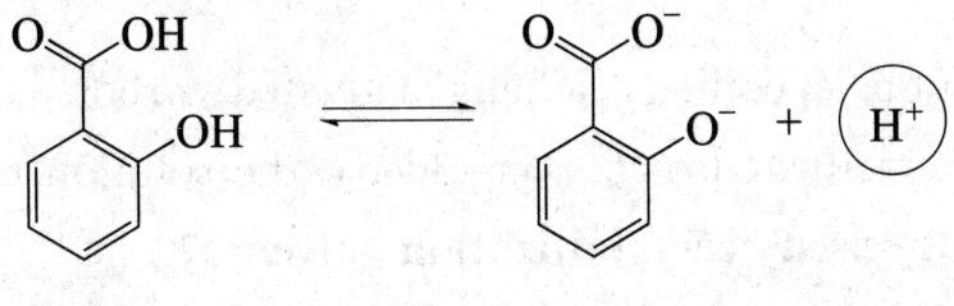

水杨酸

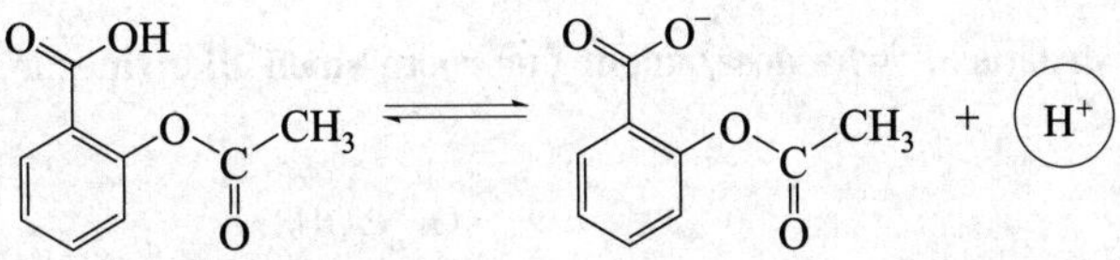

阿司匹林(2-乙酰氧基苯甲酸)

Appendix 2   Reference Answer for the Discussion Questions

Experiment 1

1. Why the activated carbon can not be added to the boiling solution when it is used as a decolorizing agent?

Answer： When the solution is boiling，adding activated carbon is easy to cause the serious bumping. Therefore，when the activated carbon is added，the solution must be slightly cold.

2. What are the commonly used recrystallization solvents?

Answer： Water，chloroform，acetone，ethyl acetate，ethanol，methanol，etc.

Experiment 2

1. In terms of structure，why dose/might our room smell like vinegar during this experiment?

Answer：

2. In terms of structure，why salicyclic and acetylsalicylic acid are considered as acids?

Answer：

Salicylic acid

Aspirin[2- (acetyloxy) -benzoic acid]

Experiment 3

1. Can acetic acid be used as an acylating agent in this preparation?

Answer： Using acetic acid as the acylating agent，the reaction time is long，many side product may also be produced，and the quality of the product is poor.

2. What are the common acylating agents?

Answer： The common acylating agents and the order of their activity is：

3. What are the common impurities of paracetamol?

Answer: The common impurities of paracetamol are:

HO—⟨ ⟩—NH—⟨ ⟩—OH

Experiment 4

1. Why not directly use aspirin and paracetamol to prepare pheniramine?

Answer: The electron density on the phenolic hydroxyl of paracetamol is low because of the conjugating of the phenolic hydroxyl to the benzene ring, which causes the weak nucleophilicity; the electron density of the phenolic oxygen atom is increased and beneficial to nucleophilic reaction after being salified, In addition, salifying can also avoid generating hydrogen chloride which can cause the hydrolysis of the resulting ester bond.

2. What are the common reagents for the preparation of carboxylic chloride from carboxylic acid?

Answer: $SOCl_2$, $(COCl)_2$, PCl_3, PCl_5.

3. Why should some pyridine be added in the preparation of acetyl salicylic chloride? What will happen if pyridine is added in excess?

Answer: Pyridine can catalize the reaction and eccelerate the reaction speed. The amout of pyridine used as a catalyst should not be excessive, otherwise the quality of the product will be affected.

Experiment 5

1. During the reaction, what are the solids precipitated at pH=7 and pH=5? What is the insoluble solid in 10 % hydrochloric acid?

Answer: The precipitated solid at pH=7 are the sulfanilamide which don't participate in the reaction; the precipitated solid at pH=5 is sulfacetamide; the insoluble material in 10 % hydrochloric acid is sulfonamidacetyl which cannot be salted out because of the absence of free aromatic primary amino groups in the structure.

2. During the reaction, it is very important to adjust pH between 12 and 13, and what will happen if alkaline is too strong or too weak?

Answer: If alkaline is too strong, the product will be hydrolyzed, so will genetate more sulfonamides but less sulfonamide diacetyl. In contrast, sulfonamidacetyl can't hydrolyze easily, so it will genetate more sulfonamidacetyl but less sulfonamide.

Experiment 6

1. When the oxidation reaction is completed, on which chemical properties dose the separation of *p*-nitrobenzoic acid from the mixture depends?

Answer: Due to the fact that *p*-nitrobenzoic acid is insoluble in water, soluble impurity in water was removed by vacuum filtration in the oxidation reaction. When the solution was adjusted to alkalinity, *p*-nitrobenzoic acid was transferred to sodium *p*-nitrobenzoic. Sodium *p*-nitrobenzoic was soluble in water. Insoluble impurity in water was removed by vacuum filtration. When the solution was adjusted to acid, sodium *p*-nitrobenzoic was retransferred to *p*-nitrobenzoic acid. The solid was got by vacuum filtration to gain final product *p*-nitrobenzoic acid.

2. Why water-free operation is needed in the esterification reaction?

Answer: Esterification reaction is reversible reaction. If water goes into the reaction system, the material will not be consumed enough. The yield will be reduced.

Experiment 7

1. What substances can be used as carriers for noble metal nanoparticles?

Answer: There are various types of substances that can be used as carriers for noble metal nanoparticles, including porous silica, metal oxides, carbon materials, metal organic frameworks (MOFs), covalent organic frameworks (COFs), and other chemical substances.

2. Regarding Pd/TB-COF catalysts, what chemical bonds are formed that allow palladium to be loaded onto TB-COF?

Answer: Palladium can be loaded onto TB-COF to obtain a supported nano catalyst Pd/TB-COF. The empty orbitals of palladium can form coordination bonds with the π electrons of imine bonds in TB-COF, thereby forming a relatively stable nano supported catalyst.

Experiment 8

1. Dissolve 0. 043 g of benzocaine in 0. 5 mL of deuterated chloroform, and use a 300 MHz nuclear magnetic resonance instrument to measure the nuclear magnetic hydrogen spectrum as shown in the following figure (indicating the chemical shift of the peak and the hydrogen number). Analyze the ^{1}H NMR spectrum of benzocaine.

Answer:

The hydrogen number corresponding to the peak with a chemical shift of 7. 8 is (1);

The hydrogen number corresponding to the peak with a chemical shift of 6. 6 is (2);

The hydrogen number corresponding to the peak with a chemical shift of 4. 3 is (4);

The hydrogen number corresponding to the peak with a chemical shift of 4. 1 is (3);

The hydrogen number corresponding to the peak with a chemical shift of 1. 3 is (4).

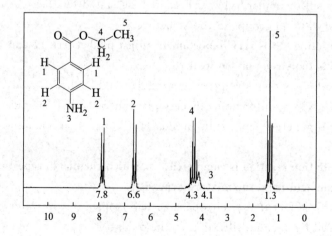

2. Provide examples to illustrate the application of hydrogenation eduction method in drug synthesis.

Answer: Catalytic hydrogenation reaction can be used for the synthesis of the anti-Alzheimer's drug donepezil hydrochloride and the antibacterial drug sulbactam.

① Synthesis of the anti Alzheimer's drug donepezil hydrochloride

② The synthesis of antibacterial drug sulbactam

Experiment 9

1. Why can the reaction be carried out in acetic acid/sodium acetate buffer when preparing 2-chloro-N-(2,6-dimethylphenyl) acetamide?

Answer: This step of the reaction uses 2,6-dimethylaniline and chloroacetyl chloride as raw materials. Due to the stronger reactivity of the reaction between chloroacetyl chloride and 2,6-dimethylaniline under weakly alkaline conditions than the reaction of acyl chloride decomposition, the acylation product can be obtained smoothly.

2. Why can chloroacetyl chloride react with 2,6-dimethylaniline and diethylamine successively?

Answer: The reactivity of the acyl chloride group and alkyl chloride atom in the chloroacetyl chloride structure is different. Therefore, by controlling the reaction conditions, chloroacetyl chloride can react with 2,6-dimethylaniline and diethylamine respectively.

Experiment 10

1. In terms of structure, why dose p-hydroxyacetophenone disssolve in potassium carbonate aqueous solution?

Answer:

2. In terms of structure, explain the reaction mechanism of Mannich condensation to dyclonine hydrochlorid.

Answer:

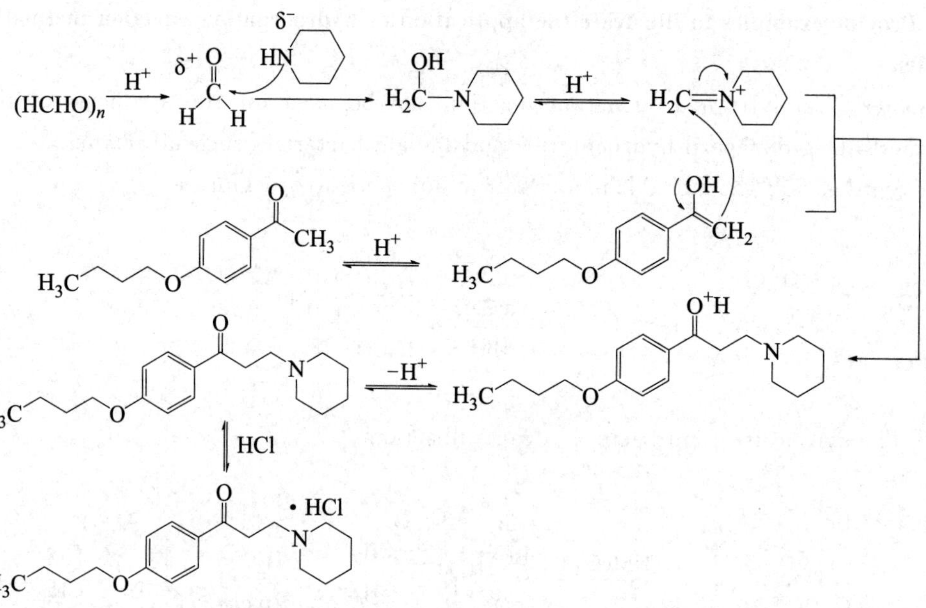

Dyclonine hydrochlorid

Experiment 11

1. What is the primary function of acetic anhydride in the reaction? Can it be replaced by other reagents?

Answer: The water generated during the reaction reacts with acetic anhydride to produce acetic acid, which is beneficial for the chemical equilibrium to shift to the right. Acetic anhydride can be replaced with other water absorbing agents.

2. What role does concentrated sulfuric acid play in the reaction? Can it be replaced by other acids?

Answer: Concentrated sulfuric acid plays a catalytic, water absorbing, and dehydration role in this reaction. Concentrated sulfuric acid can be replaced with other acids.

3. Please briefly describe the principle of Michael addition reaction.

Answer:

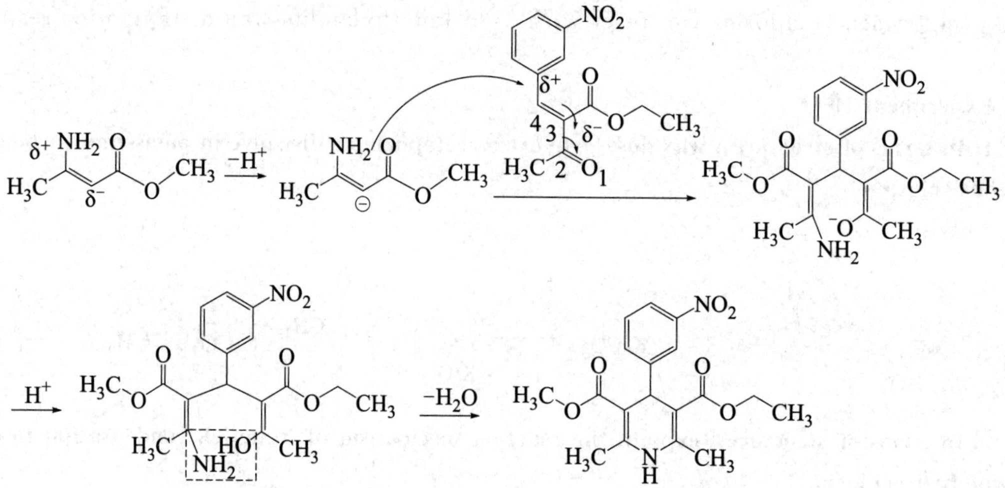

Nitrendipine

Experiment 12

1. In terms of structure, what substances can be used instead of isoamyl ethanol?

Answer: $CH_3CH_2CH_2CH_2CH_2OH$, $(CH_3)_3COH$, $CH_3CH_2CH_2CH_2OH$, etc.

2. In terms of structure, what substances are the by-product of the piperazine reaction of 6-fluoro in the condensation reaction of piperazine?

Answer:

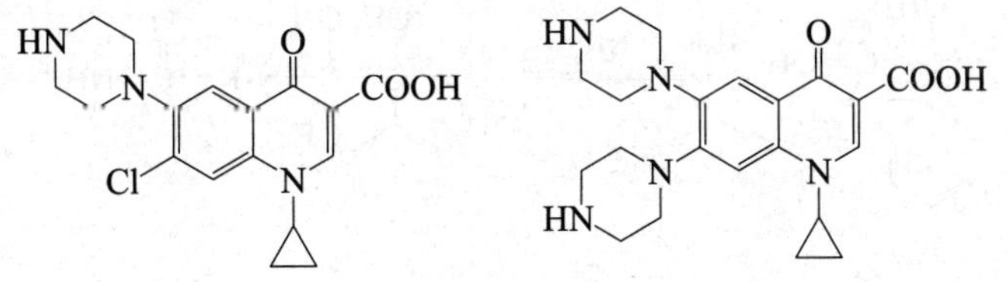

Experiment 13

1. In terms of structure, what is the mechanism of benzoin condensation catalyzed by Vitamin B_1?

Answer:

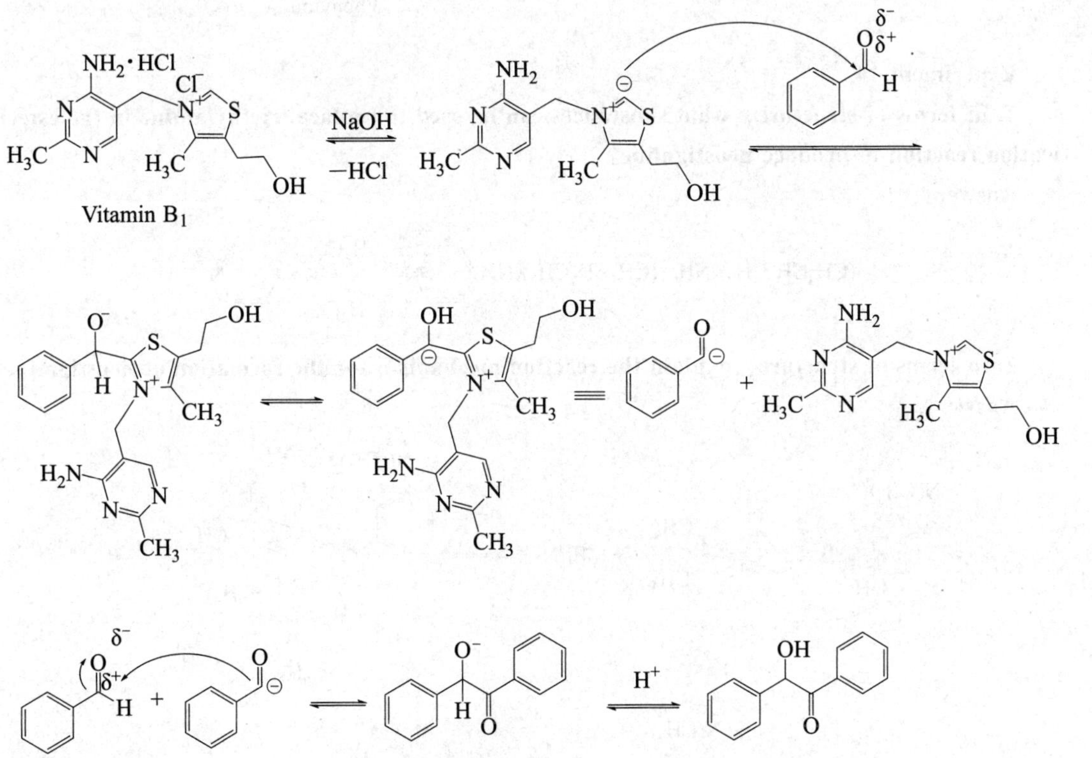

2. Can benzoin be oxidized with concentrated nitric acid in the preparation of 1,2-diphenyl-ethylene ketone?

Answer: No, strong oxidizers can destroy the chemical structure of benzoin and can not obtain the desired product.

3. In terms of structure, explain the reaction mechanism for the formation of phenytoin.

Answer:

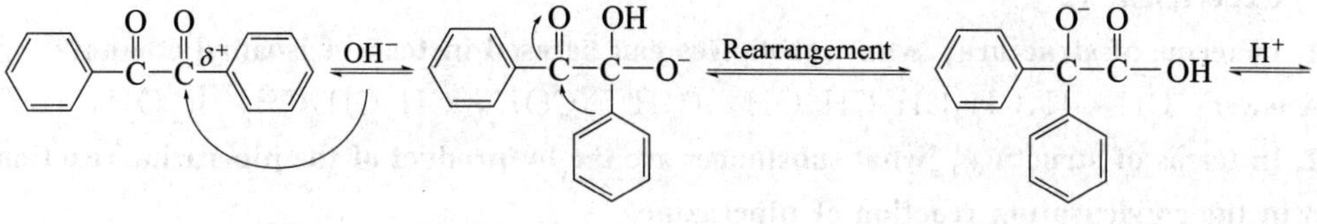

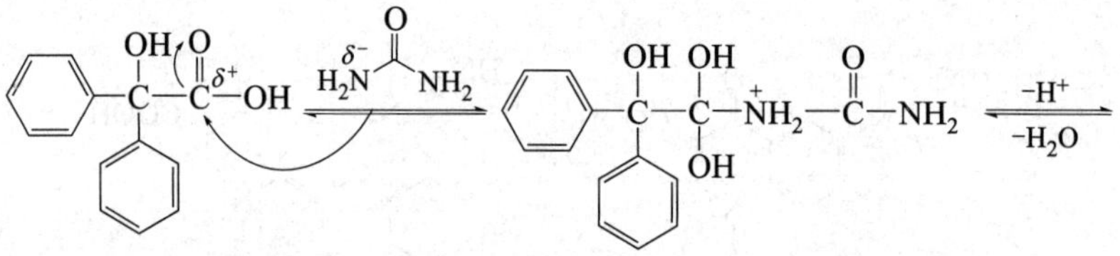

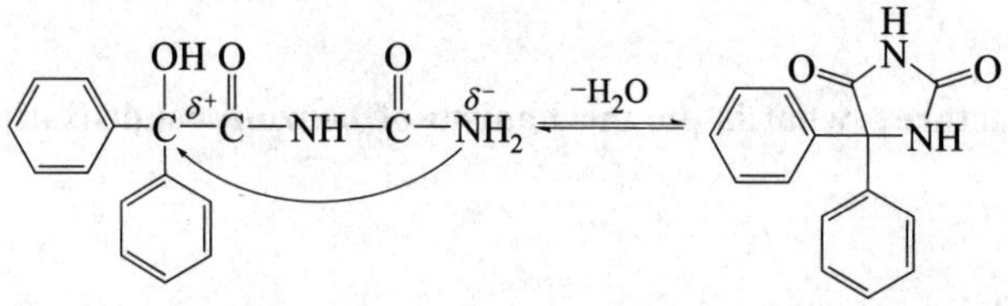

Rearrangement

Phenytoin

Experiment 14

1. In terms of structure, what substances can be used to replace triethylamine in the esterification reaction to produce neostigmine?

Answer:

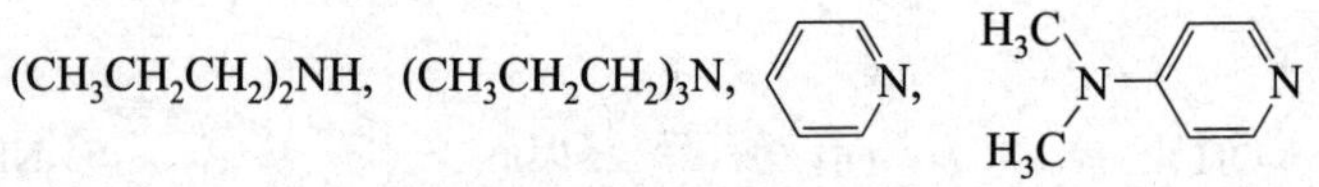

$(CH_3CH_2CH_2)_2NH$, $(CH_3CH_2CH_2)_3N$, (pyridine), (4-dimethylaminopyridine)

2. In terms of structure, explain the reaction mechanism for the formation of neostigmine.

Answer:

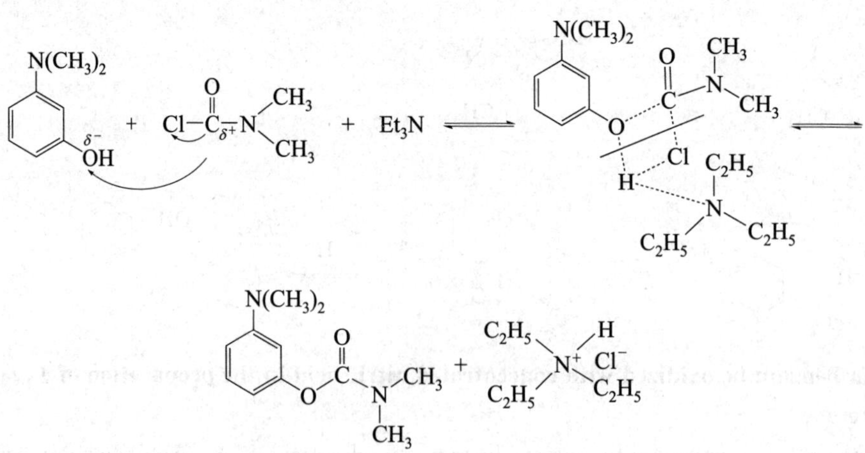

Experiment 15

1. What is the principle of the reaction between compounds 2 and 3 in this experiment?

Answer:

2. In terms of structure, what other alternatives can be used to represent the coupling reagent EDC · HCl?

Answer:

Dicyclohexylcarbodiimide(DCC)   Diisopropylcarbodiimide(DIC)

Experiment 16

1. What is the difference between the Ugi reaction and the U-3CR in this experiment?

Answer: Traditional Ugi reaction is a multi-component reaction in which the α-aminoacylamide is prepared by equivalent amounts of amine, isocyanide and carboxylic acid. In this experiment, the corresponding product is formed by chiral bicyclic imine, chiral isocyanate, and carboxylic acid.

2. Is the free radical scavenger TEMP stable? Why?

Answer: Yes, TEMPO's stable radical properties are due to the large substituents present in its structure, which prevent the radical from reacting with other molecules.

Experiment 17

1. In terms of structure, why does the quenching process of the glycosylation reaction produce gas?

Answer:

$$SnCl_4 + 2H_2O \longrightarrow H_2[SnCl_6] + HCl \uparrow$$

2. Which reagents can replace aminomethanol when removing benzoyl groups in nucleoside drug synthesis?

Answer: The removal of the benzoyl protecting group is carried out through hydrolysis reaction under alkaline conditions, and the alkaline reagents can be ammonia methanol, ammonia water, sodium methoxide, magnesium methoxide, etc.

Experiment 18

1. In terms of structure, what other reagents can be used to replace the debenzoylation reaction?

Answer:

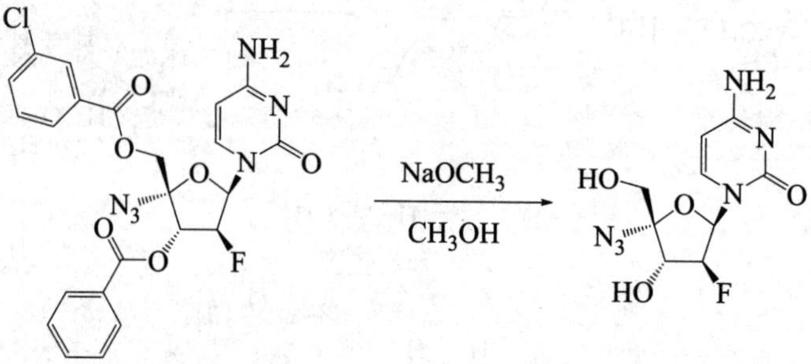

2. In terms of structure, what are the by-products of the debenzoylation reaction during the preparation of Azvudine?

Answer:

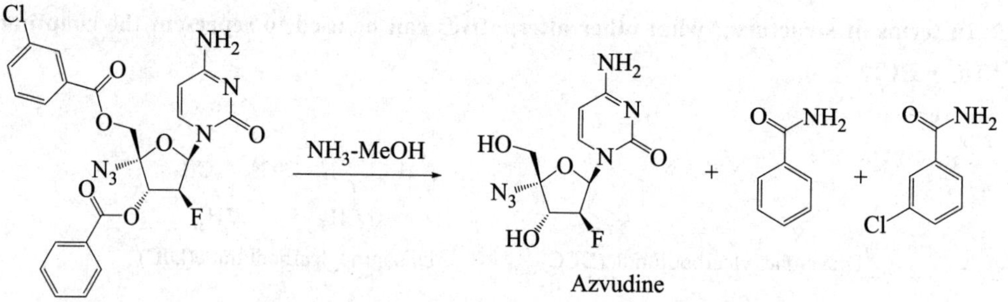

Azvudine

Experiment 19

1. What are some other methods for the synthesis of amide groups?

Answer: Amide groups can be synthesized by combining amines with carboxylic acids using a condensing agent, forming mixed anhydrides from the reaction of a carboxylic acid with an acylating agent, reacting an acyl halide with an amine, etc.

2. During the synthesis of Olverembatinib, consider what factors might affect the efficiency of the Sonogashira coupling reaction and propose possible optimization strategies.

Answer: Factors affecting the reaction include the stoichiometry of reactants, solvent selection, temperature and timing, ligand choice, and anaerobic operation. Optimization strategies include adjusting reactant ratios, selecting solvents that dissolve all components, closely monitoring the reaction with TLC, selecting catalysts and ligands for maximum catalytic activity, and maintaining an oxygen-free environment to preserve the palladium catalyst's efficacy.

附录二 思考题参考答案

实验一

1. 活性炭脱色时，为什么不能将活性炭加入到沸腾的溶液中？

答：当溶液沸腾时，加入活性炭易引起暴沸，因此，加入活性炭时，需要将溶液稍微降降温。

2. 常用的重结晶溶剂有哪些？

答：水、氯仿、丙酮、乙酸乙酯、乙醇、甲醇，等。

实验二

1. 用结构式表示，为什么反应过程中室内会有醋酸的味道？

答：

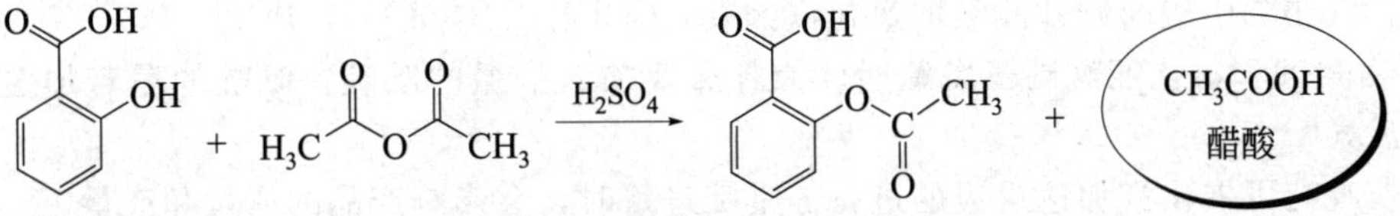

2. 用结构式表示，为什么水杨酸和阿司匹林是酸性物质？

答：

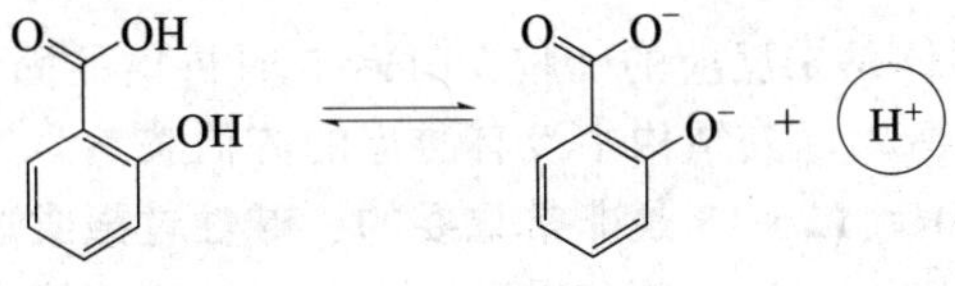

水杨酸

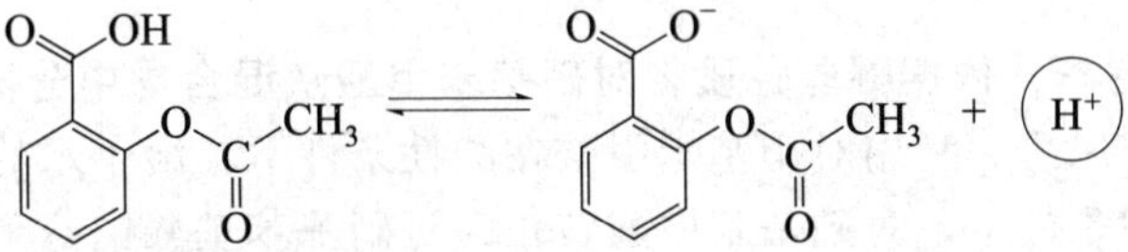

阿司匹林(2- 乙酰氧基苯甲酸)

实验三

1. 本实验中乙酸可以作为乙酰化试剂来使用吗？

答：如果本实验用乙酸作用乙酰化试剂，反应时间将被延长，并且有很多副产物生成，产品纯度很差。

2. 常用的乙酰化试剂有哪些？

答：常用的乙酰化试剂及它们的活性顺序如下：

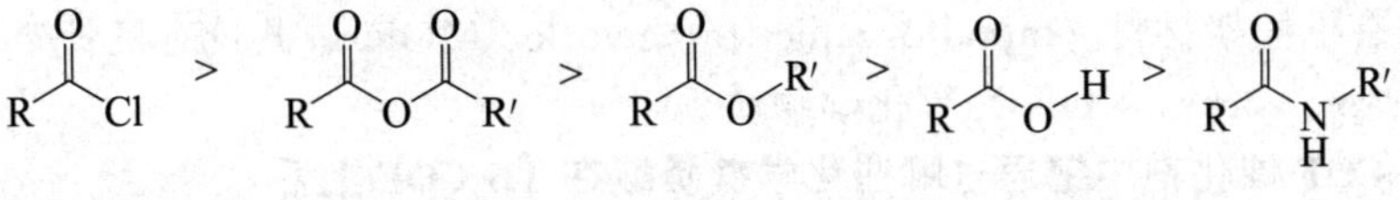

3. 合成对乙酰氨基酚时常见的杂质有哪些？

答：合成对乙酰氨基酚时常见的杂质有：

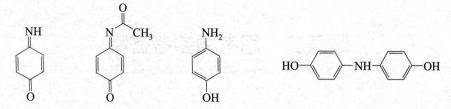

实验四

1. 为何不直接用阿司匹林和对乙酰氨基酚制备贝诺酯？

答：阿司匹林是一种低活性的芳香酸，在吡啶的催化作用下和氯化亚砜反应可生成高活性的乙酰水杨酰氯。对乙酰氨基酚上酚羟基由于与苯环的共轭作用，其亲核性较弱，当变成钠盐后，其氧上的电子密度和亲核性都会增强，另外，碱化成盐后再与乙酰水杨酰氯反应可避免生成氯化氢。

2. 由羧酸制备酰氯的常用方法有哪些？

答：常用的由羧酸制备酰氯的氯化试剂有：$SOCl_2$，$(COCl)_2$，PCl_3，PCl_5。

3. 由羧酸和氯化亚砜制备酰氯时，为什么要加入少量的吡啶？吡啶的量若加多了会发生什么后果？

答：吡啶可催化且加速反应的进行。吡啶过量时，会影响产品的质量和产量。

实验五

1. 反应过程中，pH＝7 时析出的固体是什么？pH＝5 时析出的固体是什么？在 10 % 盐酸中的不溶物是什么？

答：pH＝7 时析出的固体是未反应的磺胺；pH＝5 时析出的固体是磺胺醋酰；在 10 % 盐酸中的不溶物是磺胺双醋酰，因其结构中没有游离的芳伯胺基，故不能成盐析出。

2. 反应过程中，调节 pH＝12～13 是非常重要的，碱性过强或过弱会产生怎样的结果？

答：碱性过强，产物磺胺双醋酰、磺胺醋酰会水解，故磺胺较多；碱性过弱，磺胺双醋酰不易水解，磺胺较少。

实验六

1. 氧化反应完毕，依据哪些性质将对硝基苯甲酸从混合物中分离出来？

答：氧化反应以后，利用对硝基苯甲酸在酸性条件下不溶于水的特点，过滤留固体除去水溶性杂质；碱性条件下，对硝基苯甲酸转化为对硝基苯基酸钠溶于水，过滤要滤液除去水不溶杂质；将滤液调酸以后，对硝基苯甲酸钠游离为对硝基苯甲酸后从水中析出，过滤要固体得到产品。

2. 酯化反应为什么需无水操作？

答：酯化反应是可逆反应，如果操作过程中有水，会导致原料不能反应完全，从而导致产率下降。

实验七

1. 哪些物质可用作贵金属纳米粒子载体？

答：可用作贵金属纳米粒子载体的物质种类多样，可以是多孔二氧化硅、金属氧化物、碳材料、金属有机框架材料（metal organic framework，MOF）、共价有机骨架材料（covalent organic frameworks，COFs）等化学物质。

2. Pd/TB-COF 催化剂中钯通过哪些化学键负载在 TB-COF 上？

答：钯负载在 TB-COF 上，可获得负载型纳米催化剂 Pd/TB-COF，钯的空轨道可以和 TB-COF 中的亚胺键的 π 电子产生配位键，从而形成较为稳定的纳米负载型催化剂。

实验八

1. 将 0.043 g 苯佐卡因溶于 0.5 mL 氘代氯仿，采用 300 MHz 的核磁共振仪，测得的核磁共振氢谱如下图（标示了峰的化学位移和氢的编号），试解析苯佐卡因的核磁共振氢谱。

答案：

化学位移为 7.8 的峰对应的氢的编号为（1）；

化学位移为 6.6 的峰对应的氢的编号为（2）；

化学位移为 4.3 的峰对应的氢的编号为（4）；

化学位移为 4.1 的峰对应的氢的编号为（3）；

化学位移为 1.3 的峰对应的氢的编号为（5）。

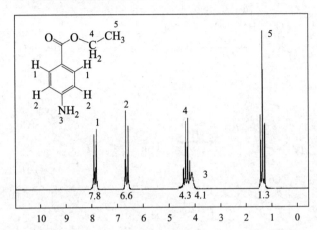

2. 举例说明加氢还原法在药物合成中的应用。

答：催化氢化反应可用于抗阿尔茨海默病药物盐酸多奈哌齐、抗菌药物舒巴坦的合成。

① 抗阿尔茨海默病药物盐酸多奈哌齐的合成

② 抗菌药物舒巴坦的合成

实验九

1. 制备 2-氯-N-(2,6-二甲苯基)乙酰胺时，为什么反应可以在醋酸/醋酸钠缓冲液中进行？

答：该步反应以 2,6-二甲基苯胺和氯乙酰氯为原料，由于在弱碱性条件下，氯乙酰氯与 2,6-二甲基苯胺反应的活泼性强于酰氯分解的反应，因此，可以顺利获得酰化产物。

2. 为什么氯乙酰氯可以先后和 2,6-二甲苯基苯胺、二乙胺发生反应？

答：氯乙酰氯结构中的酰氯基团和烷基氯原子的反应活泼性不同，因此通过控制反应条件，可以实现氯乙酰氯和 2,6-二甲基苯胺、二乙胺分别发生反应。

实验十

1. 用结构式表示，为什么对羟基苯乙酮溶于碳酸钾水溶液？

答：

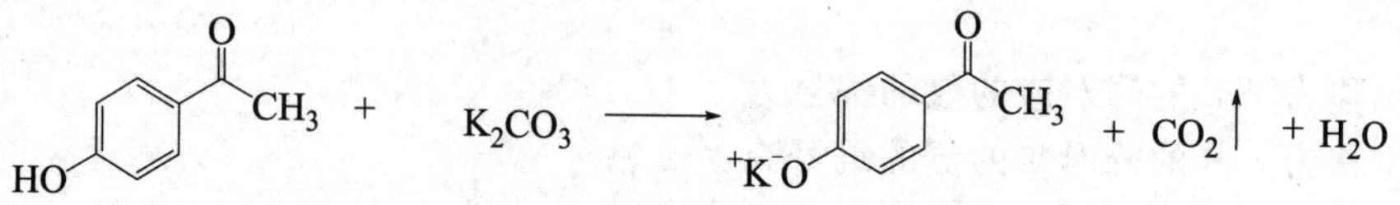

$$\text{HO-C}_6\text{H}_4\text{-COCH}_3 + K_2CO_3 \longrightarrow \text{}^+K^-\text{O-C}_6\text{H}_4\text{-COCH}_3 + CO_2\uparrow + H_2O$$

2. 用结构式表示，Mannich 缩合生成盐酸达克罗宁的反应机理。

答：

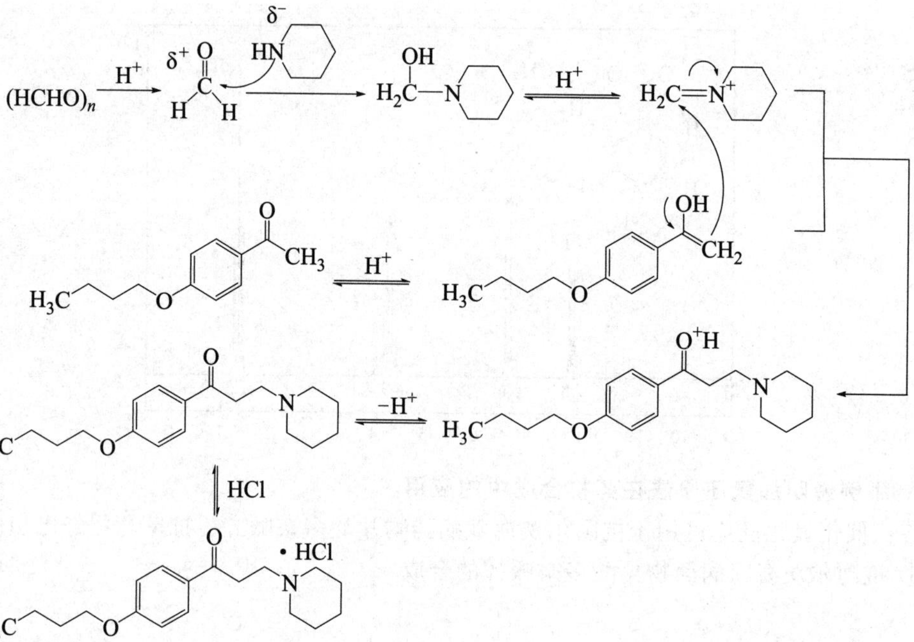

盐酸达克罗宁

实验十一

1. 乙酸酐在反应中所起的主要作用是什么？能否用其他试剂代替？

答：反应过程中生成的水与乙酸酐反应，生产醋酸，有利于化学平衡向右移。乙酸酐可以用其他的吸水试剂取代。

2. 浓硫酸在反应中起什么作用？能否用其他酸代替？

答：浓硫酸在反应中起催化、吸水和脱水作用。浓硫酸可以用其他的酸取代。

3. 简述迈克尔加成反应的原理。

答：

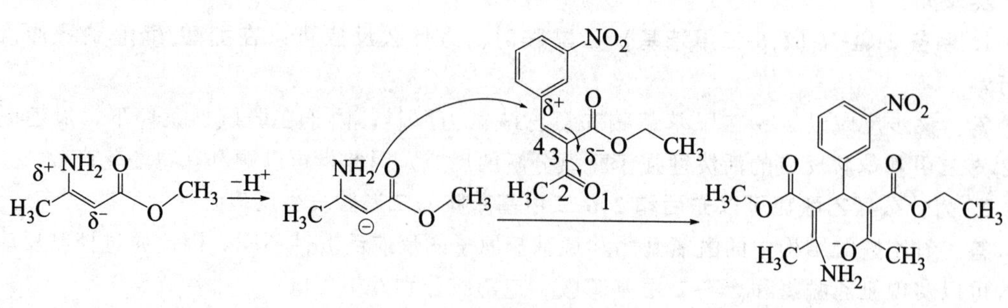

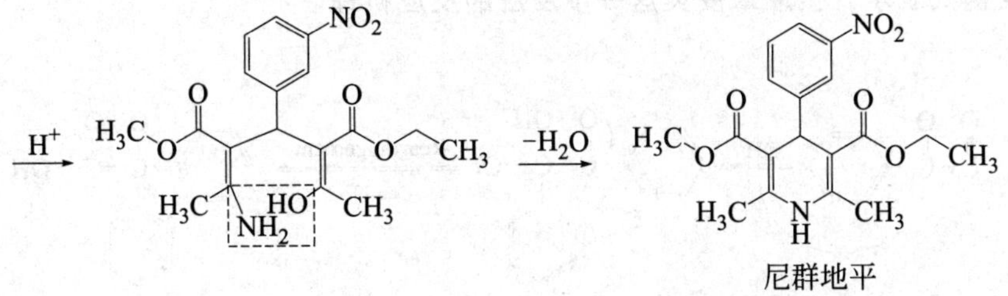

尼群地平

实验十二

1. 用结构式表示，所用异戊醇还可以用什么代替？

答：$CH_3CH_2CH_2CH_2CH_2OH$，$(CH_3)_3COH$，$CH_3CH_2CH_2CH_2OH$，等。

2. 哌嗪化反应时，6-氟发生哌嗪化副产物的结构式是什么？

答：

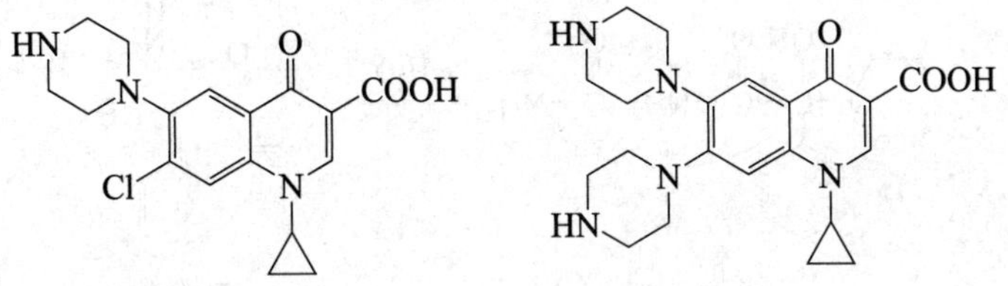

实验十三

1. 用结构式表示维生素 B₁ 催化的安息香缩合反应机理。

答：

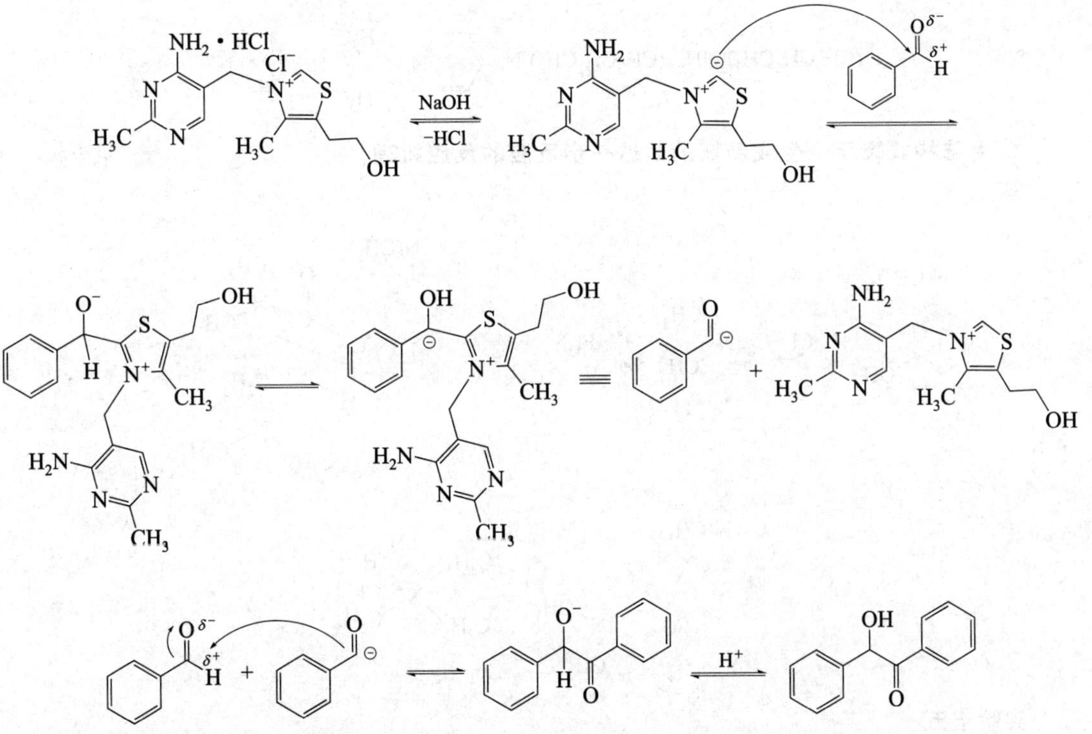

2. 制备 1,2-二苯乙二酮时，能用浓硝酸氧化安息香吗？

答：不能，强氧化剂会破坏安息香化学结构，无法获得所需要产物。

3. 用结构式表示，生成苯妥英这一步反应的反应机理。

答：

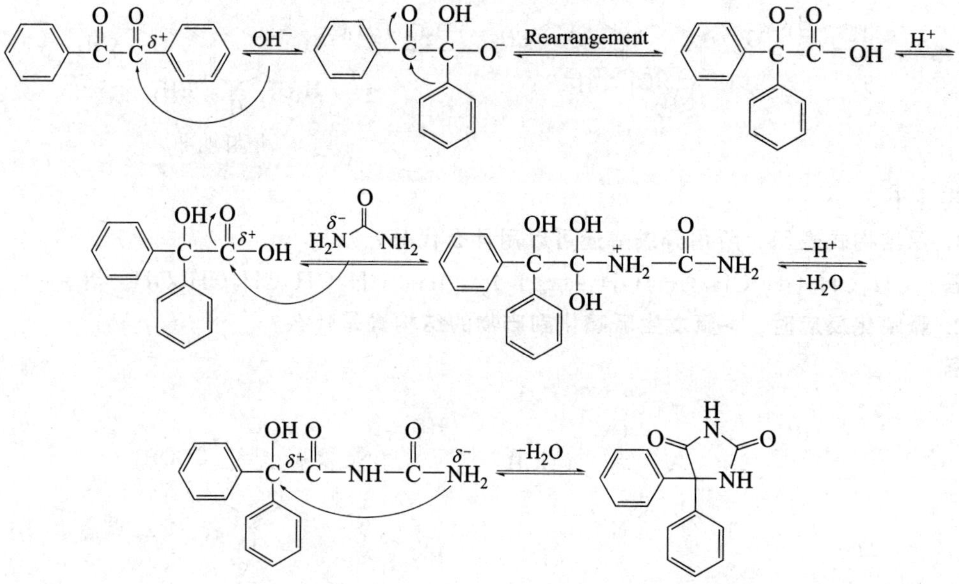

苯妥英

实验十四

1. 用结构式表示，酯化反应生成新斯的明时，可用什么物质取代三乙胺？

答：

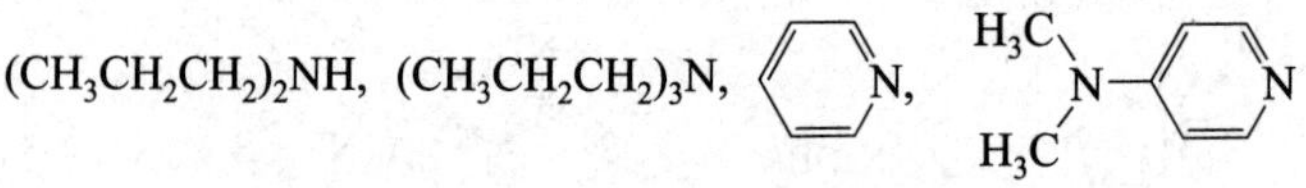

$(CH_3CH_2CH_2)_2NH$，$(CH_3CH_2CH_2)_3N$，吡啶，

2. 用结构式表示，生成新斯的明这一步反应的反应机理。

答：

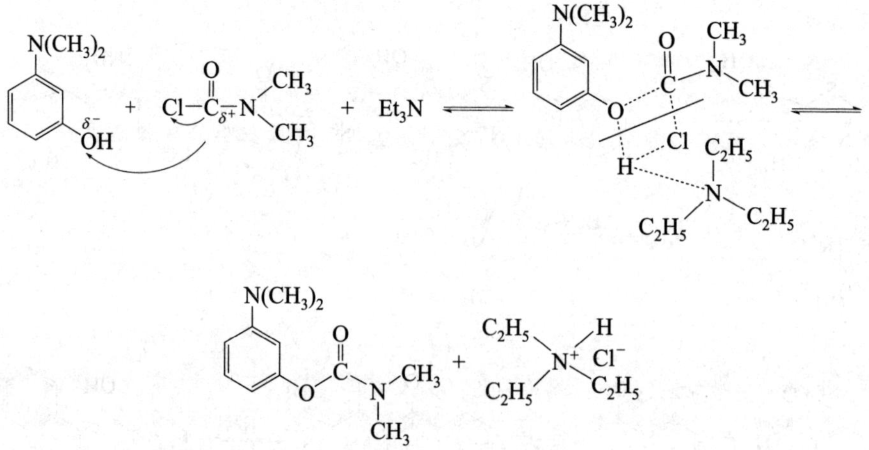

实验十五

1. 在该实验中，化合物 2 和 3 反应的原理是什么？

答：

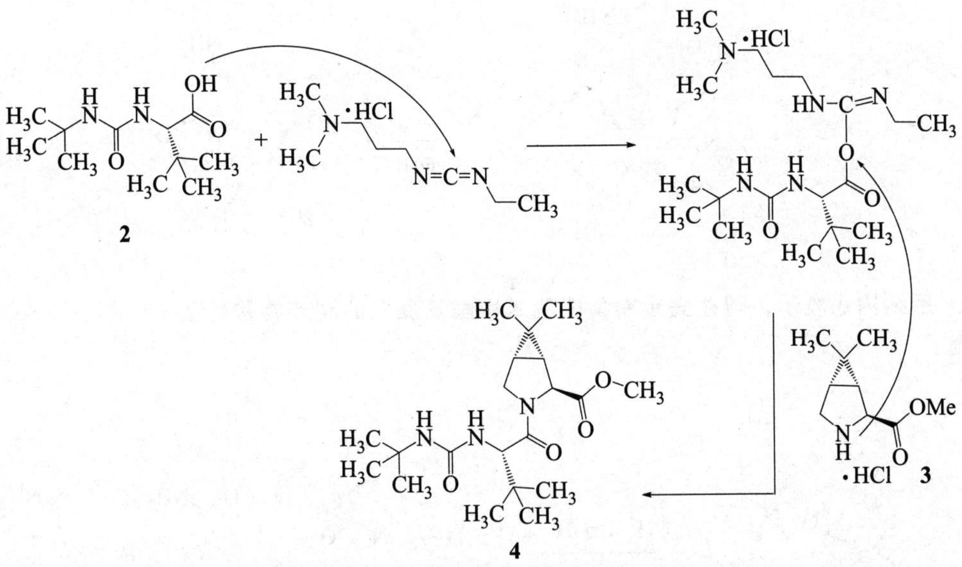

2. 用结构式表示，偶联试剂 EDC·HCl 还可以用什么代替？

答：

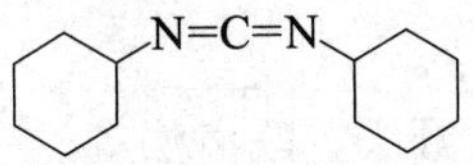

二环己基碳二亚胺（DCC） 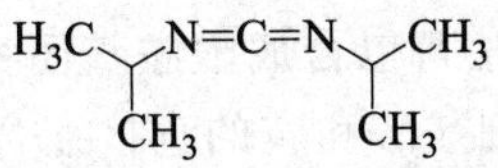　　　　二异丙基碳二亚胺（DIC）

实验十六

1. 试解释乌吉反应和本实验中乌吉三组分反应（U-3CR）的区别？

答：乌吉反应是一种多组分反应，由一分子醛或酮、一分子胺、一分子异腈以及一分子羧酸缩合生成 α-酰氨基酰胺；而本实验室中的 U-3CR 是由一分子手性双环亚胺、一分子手性异氰化物和一分子羧酸作为反应物的。

2. 自由基捕获剂 TEMP 稳定吗？为什么？

答：是的，捕获剂 TEMP 稳定。TEMPO 稳定的自由基性质是由于其自身存在的庞大的取代基，这阻碍了自由基与其它分子发生反应。

实验十七

1. 用结构式表示，在淬灭糖苷化反应的过程中，为什么有气体生成？

答：

$$SnCl_4 + 2H_2O \longrightarrow H_2[SnCl_6] + HCl\uparrow$$

2. 在核苷药物合成中，脱去苯甲酰基时，哪些试剂可替代氨甲醇？

答：脱去苯甲酰基保护基采用碱性条件下的水解反应，碱性试剂可为氨甲醇、氨水、甲醇钠、甲醇镁等。

实验十八

1. 用结构式表示，脱苯甲酰基反应还可以用什么试剂代替？

答：

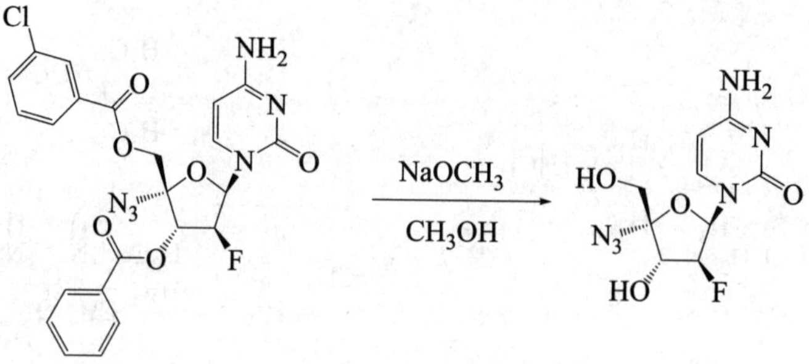

2. 用结构式表示，阿兹夫定制备时脱苯甲酰基反应的副产物是什么？

答：

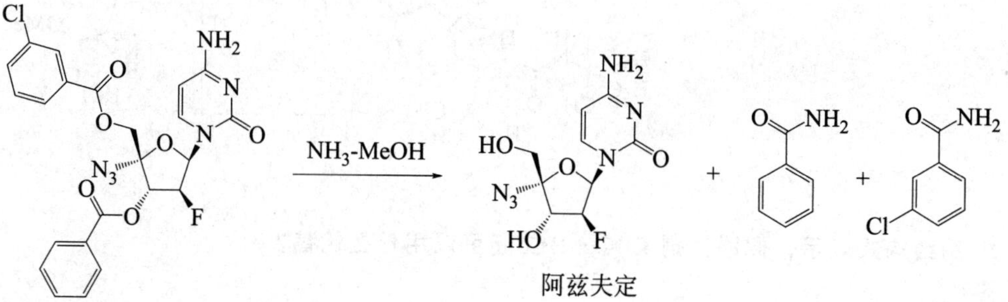

阿兹夫定

实验十九

1. 还有哪些方法可以合成酰胺基团？

答：利用缩合剂羧酸和胺的直接缩合法，混合酸酐法，酰卤法等。

2. 在合成奥雷巴替尼的过程中，考虑哪些因素可能影响 Sonogashira 偶联反应的效率，并提出可能的优化策略。

答：影响因素包括反应物的比例，溶剂的选择，反应温度和时间，配体的选择，无氧操作。优化策略：调整反应物的摩尔比例以提高效率，选择合适的溶剂以溶解所有反应物；严格控制反应温度和时间，TLC 监测反应进程；优化催化剂配体以提高催化效率；在无氧条件下进行反应，以保证钯的催化活性。

Appendix 3　Common Instruments（常用仪器）

Beaker
烧杯

Round-bottom flask
圆底烧瓶

Three-necked round-bottom
三口烧瓶

Erlenmeyer flask
锥形瓶

Filter flask
抽滤瓶

Buchner funnel
布氏漏斗

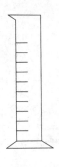

Graduated cylinder
量筒

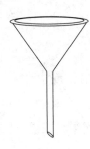

Glass funnel
玻璃漏斗

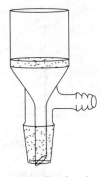

Glass filter funnel
玻璃砂芯漏斗

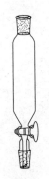

Dropping funnel
滴液漏斗

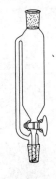

Constant pressure
dropping funnel
恒压滴液漏斗

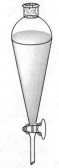

Separating funnel
分液漏斗

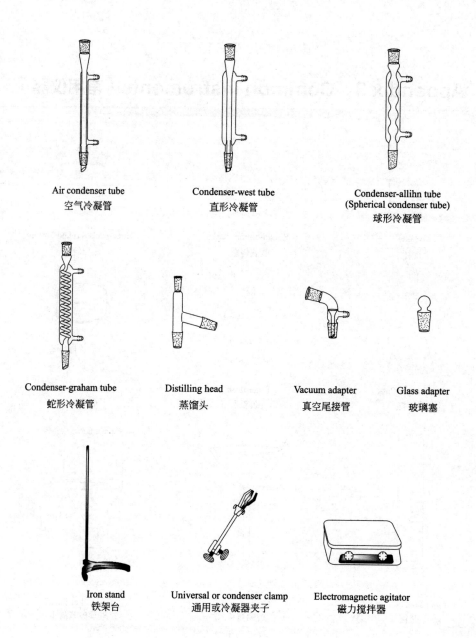

Air condenser tube
空气冷凝管

Condenser-west tube
直形冷凝管

Condenser-allihn tube
(Spherical condenser tube)
球形冷凝管

Condenser-graham tube
蛇形冷凝管

Distilling head
蒸馏头

Vacuum adapter
真空尾接管

Glass adapter
玻璃塞

Iron stand
铁架台

Universal or condenser clamp
通用或冷凝器夹子

Electromagnetic agitator
磁力搅拌器

Appendix 4 The boiling point and dielectric constant of the commonly used solvents

Solvent	b. p. /℃	Dielectric Constant[*]
N-Methylformamide	183	182. 4
Water	100	78. 4
Dimethylsulfoxide	189	46. 5
N,N-Dimethyl-formamide	153	36. 7
Methanol	64. 5	32. 7
Ethanol	78	24. 5
Acetone	56	20. 6
2-Methyl-2-propanol,t-Butanol	82. 3	12. 5
1,2-Dichloroethane	83. 5	10. 4
Dichloromethane	39. 6	8. 9
Tetrahydrofuran	66	7. 6
Ethyl acetate	78	6. 0
Chloroform	61. 2	4. 8
Diethylether	34. 4	4. 2
Toluene	110. 6	2. 4
Cyclohexane	81	1. 9
n-Heptane	98. 4	1. 9
n-Hexane	68. 7	1. 9
n-Pentane	36. 1	1. 8

* The dielectric constant is a measure of the solvent's ability to separate ions. In general, ionic compounds are more soluble in solvents with high dielectric constants.

附录四　常用溶剂的沸点和介电常数

溶剂	沸点/℃	介电常数*
N-甲基甲酰胺	183	182.4
水	100	78.4
二甲基亚砜	189	46.5
N,N-二甲基甲酰胺	153	36.7
甲醇	64.5	32.7
乙醇	78	24.5
丙酮	56	20.6
2-甲基-2-丙醇,叔丁醇	82.3	12.5
1,2-二氯乙烷	83.5	10.4
二氯甲烷	39.6	8.9
四氢呋喃	66	7.6
乙酸乙酯	78	6.0
氯仿	61.2	4.8
乙醚	34.4	4.2
甲苯	110.6	2.4
环己烷	81	1.9
n-庚烷	98.4	1.9
n-己烷	68.7	1.9
n-戊烷	36.1	1.8

* 介电常数是衡量溶剂的解离离子能力的量度,一般情况下,离子化合物更容易溶于高介电常数的溶剂中。

References（参考文献）

［1］ 尤启冬. 药物化学实验与指导（Experiment and Medicinal Chemistry）［M］. 2 版. 北京：中国医药科技出版社，2021.

［2］ 阿有梅，张红岭. 药学实验与指导（上下册）［M］. 郑州：郑州大学出版社，2015.

［3］ 木合布力·阿布力孜. 药物化学双语实验教程（Experiment of Medicinal Chemistry）［M］. 北京：科学出版社，2016.

［4］ 马玉卓. 药物化学实验（Medicinal Chemistry Experiments）（双语版）［M］. 北京：科学出版社，2016.